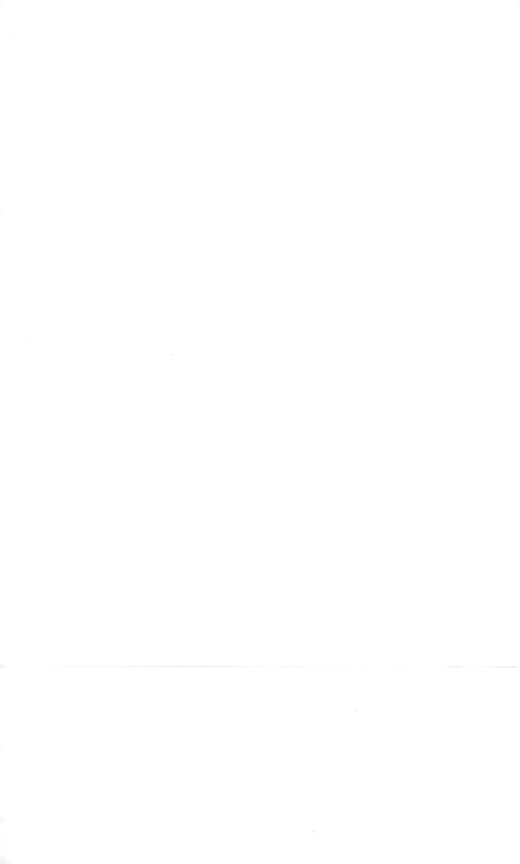

Applied Techniques in Vascular Surgery

Applied Techniques in Vascular Surgery

Edited by **Blake Forte**

New Jersey

Published by Foster Academics,
61 Van Reypen Street,
Jersey City, NJ 07306, USA
www.fosteracademics.com

Applied Techniques in Vascular Surgery
Edited by Blake Forte

© 2015 Foster Academics

International Standard Book Number: 978-1-63242-053-4 (Hardback)

Printed in the United States of America.

Contents

Preface

This book has been an outcome of determined endeavour from a group of educationists in the field. The primary objective was to involve a broad spectrum of professionals from diverse cultural background involved in the field for developing new researches. The book not only targets students but also scholars pursuing higher research for further enhancement of the theoretical and practical applications of the subject.

Vascular surgery is the field of surgery which deals with the treatment of diseases of the vascular system, or veins and arteries. This book is intended to present a concise overview on traditional open vascular surgery, endovascular surgery and pre- and post-operative handling of vascular patients. Veteran scientists and vascular surgeons from across the globe have provided valuable contributions in this book which provide descriptive and valuable information related to important topics on contemporary vascular surgery research and practice. The aim of this book is to enhance the knowledge of students and surgeons across the world and stimulate developments in this field.

It was an honour to edit such a profound book and also a challenging task to compile and examine all the relevant data for accuracy and originality. I wish to acknowledge the efforts of the contributors for submitting such brilliant and diverse chapters in the field and for endlessly working for the completion of the book. Last, but not the least; I thank my family for being a constant source of support in all my research endeavours.

Editor

Carotid Surgery

Carotid Graft Replacement of the Stenotic Carotid Artery

Igor Koncar, Nikola Ilic, Marko Dragas, Igor Banzic, Miroslav Markovic, Dusan Kostic and Lazar Davidovic

Additional information is available at the end of the chapter

1. Introduction

It is well known connection between the stroke and diseases of carotid artery (stenosis, aneurysm, kinking). In the XIX century postmortem studies showed association of ischemic brain lesions and plaque formation in carotid bifurcation [1]. Later in 1937 Egaz Moniz performed first angiography while neurologists started to consider connection between carotid and brain lesions, and very soon idea for surgical treatment was born [2]. In 1951, in Buenos Aires, Carrea performed external to internal carotid artery bypass, and published it in 1955 [3]. In the period from 1955-1975 different important cardiovascular surgical groups published their reports about surgical treatment of carotid stenosis in symptomatic patient using different reconstructive procedures. Eastcot, Pickering and Rob in 1954 reported resection of carotid bifurcation and internal to common carotid artery bypass, while DeBakey, then Row and Cooley performed carotid endarterectomy (CEA) – plaque removal instead of bypass [4, 5, 6, 7]. Afterwards idea of plaque removal instead of bypass was accepted widely, and its' efficacy in stroke prevention was later proved in multiple trials [8, 9, 10, 11, 12, 13].

Still, diverse pathologies of carotid artery were treated even before this obsession with carotid stenosis. French surgeon LeFevre used external carotid artery for flow restoration in case of traumatic lesion of internal carotid artery [14]. In the golden fifties, when carotid surgery was born, other authors reported their experience in treatment of carotid aneurysms [15, 16]. Although Dimitza used resection and reanastomosis, Beall had to use graft interposition. In this position authors were using autologous and synthetic graft with similar results; however in region susceptible to infection, autologous graft was preferred. DeBakey also reported his results in usage of graft replacement in case of carotid trauma [17]. In the beginning of treatment of carotid stenosis there were also reports of different techniques similar to those described in trauma and aneurysmatic disease. Dehnman et al treated carotid occlusion with homograft while Doyle et al used saphenous vein for treatment of carotid stenosis [18, 19]

On the other side, endarterectomy as surgical method for the treatment of stenotic arterial lesions was performed on superficial femoral artery, by Dos Santos, and later with extensive usage of Heparin it gain more success and showed its role in aorto-iliac position [20, 21]. Further experience showed its' excellent effect in focal stenotic lesions in vessels with large-caliber and high-flow rate. In everyday clinical practice this technique has proved efficient in patients with localized disease limited to the distal aorta or proximal iliac arteries and distal common femoral artery obstructing deep femoral artery orifice (profundoplasty) [22, 23, 24]. On the contrary in extensive atherosclerotic pattern that are more frequent in clinical practice, endarterectomy is technically demanding with poor long term results [25]. Later trough history, short lesions were preferably treated by endovascular means, leaving bypass reconstruction for longer ones, while isolated endarterectomy is becoming almost forgotten except in carotid bifurcation. It is rarely recognized in the literature that in some, not frequent, situations endarterectomy in stenotic carotid artery is not possible or it might be jeopardized. What are modes of reconstruction of carotid artery when CEA fails or is not possible? If bypass or graft replacement is alternative in peripheral occlusive disease, should we apply it in carotid position as well in situations when extensive disease is encountered or technical challenge happens?

2. Aim of the chapter

The aim of this chapter is to show results and experience of a single high volume center in usage of synthetic graft in the treatment of extensive carotid atherosclerotic disease and to analyze published results related to this topic.

3. Material and methods

Clinic for Vascular and Endovascular Surgery of the Serbian Clinical Center is located in Belgrade, Serbia, and it was part of the Second surgical clinic, the cradle of cardiovascular medicine in the former Yugoslavia. First vascular procedures were performed in its' facilities in the sixties (1966) by outstanding pioneers of this, in that time, new branch of surgery – V. Stojanovic and B. Vujadinovic. Figure 1 (A and B). Further development of this institution was supported by the fact that it becomes educational and referral center. Intensive cooperation with leading world centers of excellence, sending its practitioners for education and organizing demonstrational operations in own facilities contributed to popularization and development of cardiovascular surgery in the former Yugoslavia, Balkans and Eastern Europe with consequent progress in treatment of cardiovascular patients in this institution. Later S.Lotina, (Figure 1 - C) successor of Stojanovic and Vujadinovic, has significant role in development of vascular surgery in this institution, since he struggled for segmentation of cardiovascular surgery in the late eighties and middle nineties and eventually achieved expansion of independent vascular department with surgeons and angiologists dedicated to this field. Later, Lazar Davidovic, (Figure 1 - D) one of his pupils, becomes new leader of this department accomplished to improve it to the level of the clinic. After finishing his education with fellowship at Pitié-Salpêtrière hospital in Paris, under the service of Prof Eduard Kieffer, where he improved his experience in aortic and carotid surgery, adopting eversion technique, L. Davidovic brought new modern perspectives in the diagnosis and treatment of vascular patients not only in this institution but rather in the whole country of Serbia. Since then the number of carotid and aortic procedures is annually increasing in this institution reaching almost 600 carotid and almost 500 aortic in the year 2011, with sensible and gradually introduction of endovascular procedures (carotid, peripheral stenting and endovascular repair of aortic pathology) according to published results, guidelines recommendation and available financial support of national health care system.

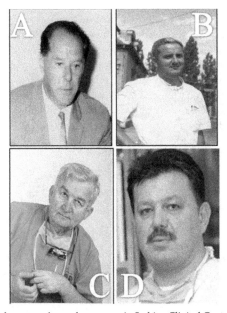

Figure 1. Leaders of development of vascular surgery in Serbian Clinical Centre in last 60 years. A. Vojislav Stojanovic (1955-1971) B. Borislav Vujadinovic (1971-1985) C. Slobodan Lotina (1985-2002) D. Lazar Davidovic (2002- still leading Clinic for Vascular and Endovascular Surgery)

In the period from January 2003 to October 2006, at the Clinic for Vascular and Endovascular Surgery of the Serbian Clinical Centre, 1250 procedures due to carotid artery stenosis in 1127 patients were performed. Carotid stenosis was repaired by eversion or conventional endarterectomy (CEA) and synthetic graft (Dacron®) interposition in 987 (78, 96 %), 205 (16, 4 %) and 58 (4, 64 %) patients respectively. We retrospectively analyzed prospectively gathered data related to the subgroup of patients operated with graft replacement.

Indications for conventional EA with usage of protective intraluminal shunt were contralateral occlusion, recent stroke or transitory ischemic attack and intraoperative stump pressure below 40mmHg. These patients were excluded from this analysis. Other patients were operated with eversion technique. Eversion EA was performed in the same manner as described elsewhere in the literature [26].

Indications for graft replacement (GR) were: extensive atherosclerotic disease proximal and/or distal to carotid bifurcation revealed intraoperatively during dissection or preoperatively by means of ultrasound, digital subtraction angiography (Figure 3.) or multidetector computed tomography; long segment of thrombotic surface after EA; bad quality of arterial wall after EA; inadequate end of the endarterectomy cleavage; any other technical problem that could endanger the success of procedure. Decision for GR was made by operating surgeon.

GR was performed after complete resection of carotid bifurcation and its removal. Dacron graft of 6 or 8 mm in diameter was used depending on the ICA and CCA diameter. Initially anastomosis between the graft and ICA was made, in the continuous fashion, "parachute" technique, with Prolene 6-0 suture. Upon finishing the anastomosis clamp was removed proximaly on the synthetic graft in order to verify anastomotic compatibility. Afterwards proximal anastomosis between CCA and synthetic graft was sutured with Prolene 5-0 in the same fashion. Flushing and air removal is of outmost importance before declamping since there is in-line flow directly to endocranial vascular bed without any patent branch. Reattachment of ECA was performed selectively according to its quality, position and already spent time for GR (Figure 2 and 3.).

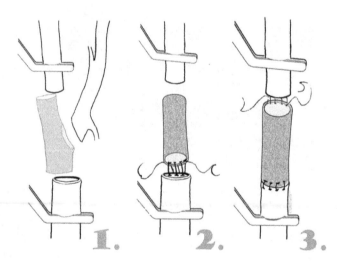

Figure 2. Schematic presentation of carotid graft replacement. A. Resection of carotid bifurcation B. Suturing distal anastomosis C. Suturing proximal anastomosis

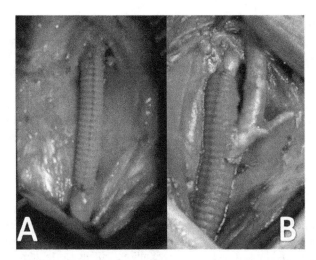

Figure 3. Intraoperative image of final graft reconstruction A. Dacron graft interposition B. Dacron graft interposition with reimplanted external carotid artery

In this period of time (2003-2006) cervical plexus block was introduced for carotid surgery in our institution, and consequently we changed the indications for conventional endarterectomy and shunt usage performing it only in case of neurological deterioration of the patient during carotid cross clamping. However patients treated with conventional EA with extensive atherosclerotic disease were not analyzed in this paper and GR was performed without usage of the intraluminal shunt.

Among 1045 procedures performed in 956 patients there were 987 (94, 45%) treated with eversion EA and 58 (5, 55%) with GR. After excluding patients treated with conventional and eversion EA, we retrospectively analyzed preoperative, intraoperative and postoperative data of the patients treated with GR in order to investigate results of this alternative procedure and to try to define optimal indications for its' usage. After analyzing initial results deeper investigation was performed by dividing group of patients treated with GR in two groups according to the indication and decision to perform GR:

Group A, when decision to perform GR was made according to the ultrasonography exam and intraoperative findings before any attempted EA;

Group B when GR was made after failed EA as a bailout procedure.

In the preoperative data we analyzed age, sex, co-morbid conditions and preoperative ultrasound descriptions. All patients were preoperatively examined by ultrasonography means, describing quality and length of the plaque. All exams were made by experienced ultrasonographer. The quality of plaque was described as lipid, fibrous or calcified with or without present ulceration. The length of the plaque was defined as the longitudinal extent of the plaque narrowing arterial lumen for 30% and more. Plaques longer than 4cm were named as long.

After removing atherosclerotic plaque from internal carotid artery (ICA) and common carotid artery (CCA) its' quality (morphology) and length were assessed too. From intraoperative data we used the intraoperative length of atherosclerotic disease, reasons to perform GR (before any attempt to perform eversion or after attempted eversion), cross clamping time and restoration of external carotid artery flow.

Postoperative data were related to the neurological outcome and mortality rate as well as early surgical (hemorrhage, cranial nerve lesions, and wound infection) and cardiac complications. All patients were followed for one month and yearly thereafter with clinical and ultrasound examination.

4. Results

Among treated patients significant number was symptomatic - 30 (51, 72 %) patients with previous transitory ischemic attack (12 – 40%), ocular symptoms (2 – 6, 66%) or stroke (16 – 53, 33%). Demographic characteristics of the patients and symptoms distribution were presented in the Table 1. There was no significant difference in terms of co-morbid conditions between the groups.

Characteristic/ Group	Graft replacement N (%)	Subgroup A/B N (%)
Number of patients	58 (100)	40 (68.96) / 18(31.04)
Age	65.55	66.8 / 64.3
Male	50 (86.2)	34 (85) / 16 (88.88)
Arterial Hypertension	48 (82.75)	35 (87.5) / 13 (72.22)
Smoking	40 (68.96)	28 (70) / 12 (66.66)
Obesity	10 (27.24)	7 (17.5) / 3 (16.66)
Diabetes	32 (55.17)	23 (57.5) / 9 (50)
Angina pectoris	24 (41.3)	18 (45) / 6 (33.33)
Myocardial infarction	15 (25.86)	11 (27.5) / 4 (22.22)
Aortic disease	5 (8.62)	4 (10) / 1 (5.55)
Peripheral disease	9 (15.51)	6 (15) / 3 (16.66)
Previous CABG	8 (13.79)	5 (12.5) / 3 (16.66)
Previous aortic procedures	2 (3.44)	2 (5) / 0
Previous peripheral procedures	0	0
Symptoms		
Asymptomatic	28 (48.27)	
Symptomatic	30 (51.73)	
Transitory ischemic attack	12 (40)	
Ocular symptoms	2 (6.66)	
Stroke	16 (53.33)	

Table 1. Demographic characteristic of the patients and preoperative symptoms

There was no significant difference between ultrasonography and intraoperative findings in the group A. There was significant difference between ultrasonography and intraoperative findings of the plaque length on the CCA and ICA among patients of group B. There was significant number of patients with plaque length of 4cm and more in the CCA, described in the ultrasonography exam and found intraoperatively. Tables 2 and 3

Plaque morphology	Ultrasonography	Intraoperative findings	P
	Group A (40 patients)	Group A (40 patients)	
Fibrous plaque/ with ulceration	7 (17.5%) / tructio5 (12.5%)	5 (12.5%) / 0	P > 0.05
Lipid plaque/ with ulceration	5 (12.5%) / 1 (2.5 %)	9 (22.5%) / 1 (2.5 %)	P > 0.05
Calcified plaque/ with ulceration	6 (15%) / 19 (48%)	11 (27.5%) / 14 (34.5%)	P < 0.05
CCA plaque length> 4cm	19 (48%)	22 (55%)	P > 0.05
ICA plaque length> 4cm	12 (29.5%)	19 (48%)	P > 0.05

Table 2. Comparison of ultrasonography and intraoperative findings in the patients of the group A

Plaque morphology	Ultrasonography	Intraoperative findings	P
	Group B (18 patients)	Group B (18 patients)	
Fibrous plaque/ with ulceration	4 (22.2%) / 1 (5.06)	2 (11%) / 0	P > 0.05
Lipid plaque/ with ulceration	2 (11%) / 0	2 (11%) / 1 (5.06%)	P > 0.05
Calcified plaque/ with ulceration	3 (16.6 %) / 8 (44.44%)	6 (33.33 %) / 7 (38.88%)	P > 0.05
CCA plaque length> 4cm	6 (33.3%)	10 (55.55%)	P > 0.05
ICA plaque length> 4cm	0	3 (16.66%)	**P<0.05**

Table 3. Comparison of ultrasonography and intraoperative findings in the patients of the group B

Intraoperative data were presented in the table 4. Among 58 patients, 22 (37.93%) were operated in conditions of general anesthesia and 26 (62.07%) under cervical plexus block. Mean cross clamping time was measured and presented in Figure 2. There was significantly longer cross clamping time when GR was made after attempted EA. ECA flow restoration was made in 9 (15.6%) patients with intraoperative decision of the operating surgeon according to the quality of ECA, its' position related to the implanted graft and elapsed time of the procedure. Reimplantation of ECA did not influence on neurological complication rate.

Early postoperative recovery was uneventful in 36 patients (95%). Early death was reported in 2 patients (5%), due to fatal stroke in the early postoperative time. More one patient had transitory ischemic attack (2,5%) and one had minor stroke (2,5%). Total rate of neurological complications is 7.5%. Comparison of the neurological complications between the groups found higher rates when EA was unsuccessful and GR performed as a bail out procedure. Permanent cranial nerve injuries were reported in 1 patient (2.5%). There was neither early myocardial infarction nor death based on any other cause in this series.

Patients were followed by means of ultrasonography one month after the procedure and yearly thereafter. Mean follow up time was 32 months. Two patients were lost from follow up while 4 patients (10.52%) died during this period of time. Restenosis of less than 75% was reported in 2 patients (5.26%), restenosis of 75-99% was found in 1 patient (2.78%) successfully treated with carotid stenting (Figure 5). In one patient total occlusion of reconstructed artery was revealed with no neurological symptoms.

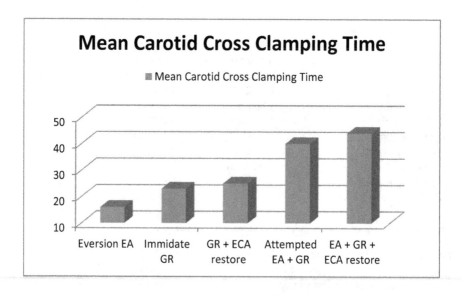

Figure 4. Mean cross clamping time

Author	Number of patients	Graft material	Extensive disease	Other indications	Irradiational arteritis	Stroke rate	Patency rate	Mean follow up (months)
W.Moore/ Dorafshar [47]	41	PTFE 31 GSV 10	9 (22.5%)	Restenosis 28 (68.29%) Aneurysm 3 (7.31%) Glomus Tu 2 (4.87%) Kinking 1 (2.43%) Dissection 1 (2.43%)	5 (12.19%)	4,9 %	PTFE 90 % GSV 80%	50
Camiade [46]	110	PTFE	45 (41%)	Restenosis 18 (16.4%) Kinking 29 (26.4%)	7 (6.4%)	0.9 %	95%	22
Lauder [39]	50	GSV	22 (44%)	Kinking 14 (28%)	-	4 %	83%	36/60
Veldeniz [42]	51	Dacron	27 (53%)	-	-	1.9%	96%	36
Brancherau [43]	212	GSV	161(76%)	Restenosis 12 (5.6%) Aneurysm 9 (4.24%) Kinking 18 (8.49%)	-	5%	96%	104
Cormier [38]	62	PTFE	54 (87%)	-	-	5 %	97%	23
Sise MJ [40]	26	PTFE	Technical problem 9 (34.61%) Carotid thrombosis 2 (7.69%)	Restenosis 9 (34.61%) Aneurysm 6 (23.07%)	-	0%	96%	36
Fabiani [45]	51	GSV	Prospective comparative trial compared CEA with GSV interposition			0%	2% Restenosis	52

Table 4. Published results since 1979

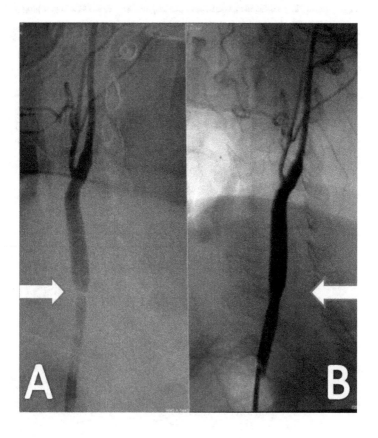

Figure 5. Restenosis at the proximal anastomosis (A) resolved with carotid stenting (B)

5. Discussion

There is no doubt that, over all, endarterectomy is the optimal technique for surgical repair of carotid stenosis. This is the only location where EA is the preferable method nowadays. Choice of EA (conventional or eversion) might cause some discussion between vascular surgeons however the last meta-analysis gave slight advantage to eversion, which was also shown by randomized trial in our institution [27, 28]. Previous Meta analysis showed no difference between the two techniques [27]. The former includes a standard longitudinal carotid arteriotomy with or without patch angioplasty, whereas the second encompasses an oblique transection and eversion of the internal carotid artery and its' reimplantation into the common carotid artery [29, 30, 31]. Regarding the carotid artery closure after conventional EA, carotid patch angioplasty is preferable to primary closure [32].

Conventional EA requires usage of graft material that is extending procedure and expose patient to the risk of infection [33]. Eversion EA on the other side does not provide sufficient insight in to the complete endarterectomized surface in the zone at the end of the removed atherosclerotic plaque. Also preparing carotid bifurcation for eversion EA requires its complete deliberation from surrounding tissue which might increase the risk of distal embolizations. Elongated internal carotid artery makes patch suturing more complex while shunt placement in these situations is raising the difficulties. Redundant ICA might simplify eversion EA on the other side. Both of these techniques are related to some advantages and disadvantages including surgeons' familiarity as a specific one. Both of the techniques requires volume of patients in order to achieve good results what might influence the diverse adoption between the teams. According to one multinational registry there is difference in the usage rate of these techniques – in eight European countries EA was performed without patch (34%), with patch (40%) or with eversion (26%). Finally, guidelines of the most important and leading societies are leaving the choice between the two techniques to the operating surgeon [32, 34]. Does it mean that any procedure that removes atherosclerotic plaque from carotid bifurcation and restores flow in a short and long term would be effective in stroke prevention? The similar theory said M.E. DeBakey sixty years ago before his first carotid procedure. DeBakey reasoned that, since endarterectomy and graft replacement in other arteries could be performed, the carotid artery should not be an exception [35].

Carotid stenosis is most frequently localized at the carotid bifurcation leaving proximal and distal segments free from disease providing suitable conditions for endarterectomy. Extension of the atherosclerotic process towards proximally or distally might make endarterectomy cumbersome and risky, while multiple severe atherosclerotic changes at different levels of supra-aortic branches require anatomical or extra-anatomical bypass procedure. Group of patients analyzed in this chapter belongs somewhere between these two patterns of carotid disease – not enough extensive for anatomical bypass through sternotomy while substantially extensive and challenging for eversion EA.

From technical point of view atherosclerotic process that extends proximally and/or distally aggravates endarterectomy jeopardizing the procedure. Initial problem is *carotid clamping*. It is necessary to extensively dissect internal and common carotid artery in order to provide safe clamping. Clamping at inadequate location of diseased artery might cause plaque rupture with consequent prone to thrombosis causing perioperative embolizations. Also, clamping at inadequate location could cause incomplete EA causing thrombosis especially at the internal carotid artery location. Preventing incomplete EA in this situation requires additional dissection which is more challenging during clamped and transected carotid artery, it prolongs cross clamping time and might stress inexperienced surgeon provoking other mistakes. Reaching healthy zone is important likewise for shunt users in order to prevent placing a shunt through atherosclerotique plaque inducing distal embolizations. Once reaching the conform clamping zone we are faced with technicaly demanding extensive EA. In case of eversion technique problems are visualization of the end of the plaque zone, adequate flushing of the left surface and removal of small residual intimal particles that are prone to mobilization causing distal embolizations [36]. Extensive dissection of internal carotid artery and its deliberation from surrounding tissue facilitate its eversion. On the contrary, common carotid artery is even more difficult to evert through the whole circumference since the posterior wall is fixed with the external carotid artery. Due to that flexibility of common carotid artery depends on deliberation of external carotid artery from surrounding tissue too. In case of extensive athersoclerosis of common carotid artery and average to minimal process on internal carotid artery it is advisable to transect common carotid artery proximal from its' bifurcation instead of transecting internal carotid artery. This techniqe provides easier EA of common carotid artery in a longer segment [7]. Another technical possibility to deal with extensive atherosclerotic disease in common carotid artery could be semi closed endarterectomy by using Vollmars rings. Finally, for those who preffer conventional technique the very process of EA is quite easier with adequate visualisation of the end of the plaque zone, however, finally the Achille heel of this method is long patch anastomosis that is technicaly demanding and more prone to neointimal hyperplasia or false aneurysm. Anastomotic bleeding on the long patch is another technical difficutly especialy when using intraluminal shunt. Upon removing the shunt, brain perfusion is reduced until complete haemostasis is provided making declamping safe. Loosing time on resolving anastomotic bleeding could cause ishemic brain injury. Overcoming all these technical difficulties does not guarantee sucess since long endarterectomy is leaving long thrombogenic surface prone to in situ thrombosis or distal embolizations jeopardizing the results of the procedure regardless to excellent surgical technique.

All these difficulties were encountered in peripheral vascular surgery inducing usage of different conduits in the reconstructive bypass procedures; similar was done in carotid surgery although less frequently. Bypass in this location could have a good long term potential since it is connecting two healthy arteries with high blood flow and loaded recipient vascular bed, like cerebral, which is inducing low resistance. Still low number of publications is describing this technique in the last 30 years with usage of different conduits.

Consequently in the two most respected guidelines for treatment of carotid stenosis this option is not mentioned. However a short review of the published data related to this technique is given below with some technical remarks from the authors of this chapter.

In 1979 M.E.Debakey published his experience in usage of synthetic graft for repair of carotid artery injury [37]. In the same year Cormier and all started to use this type of reconstruction reporting their experience eight years later [38]. Among 62 treated patients 54 (87%) were treated due to extensive atherosclerotic disease, with 5% stroke rate and 97% patency in the 23 months long term follow up. Later, different types of reconstruction were reported using various conduits. Camiade and all used PTFE graft suture with side to end proximally and end to side anastomosis distaly [39]. This technique minimizes dissection of carotid bifurcation and preserves patency of external carotid artery. Authors performed this procedure in 110 patients, indicated it in case of extensive atherosclerotic disease in 45 (41%), while using it also for reconstruction in case od restenosis (16.4%) or kinking (26.4%). There were some other authors reporting usage PTFE graft with similar patency of 95-97% in the long term [40, 41]. The only author that used Dacron graft was Valdeniz with results comparable to those published with PTFE [42]. Autologous saphenous vein was also reported by various authors, some of them complaining on high restenosis rate. French authors are reporting good early and long term results [43, 44, 45]. In 212 patients treated due to extensive atherosclerotic disease (76%), restenosis (5.6%), kinking (8.49%) and aneurysm (4.24%) they reported 5% stroke rate and 96% patency after average 104 months of follow up. On the other side according to the Leicester group saphenous vein is prone to early restenosis in this position even though they performed different anastomotic techniques [46]. According to the diameter of the vein graft and common carotid artery they located anastomosis at the lateral wall of common carotid artery, at the origin of internal carotid artery or at the origin of external carotid artery after its' exclusion. After average follow up of 60 months patency rate was 83% with significant incidence of restenosis. According to opinion of the authors of this chapter vein graft could be perfect for this procedure, however one might expect misfit of the calibers. Additionally harvesting this graft could be time consuming if so if the graft replacement is performed as a bailout procedure it might prolong cross clamping time and procedure. It is not convenient for carotid procedures performed in cervical plexus block and finally saphenous vein is important conduit for coronary revascularization and should be preserved for that occasion as well. This conduit could be unavailable in patients with varicose syndrome and previous coronary revascularization. Latest publication is from W. Moore reporting 17 years of experience using both synthetic and saphenous vein grafts with satisfying results [47]. 31 PTFE and 10 saphenous grafts were followed for 50 months with patency of 90% and 80%, respectively. Carotid graft replacement is already proved procedure in some other pathology like carotid artery aneurysm and restenosis [48, 49].

Summarized published data show 613 carotid procedures where bifurcation was reconstructed with GR. In all these publications the most frequent indication for graft usage was extensive atherosclerotic disease with involvement of common or distal internal carotid artery – 328 procedures (53.5%). Other indications were carotid recurrent stenosis, technical failure of attempted EA, stenosis after radiation therapy, carotid aneurysm and carotid stenosis associated with kinking. Among 613 carotid stenosis treated with GR, 290 (47,3%) procedures were performed with PTFE graft, 272 (44,37%) with saphenous graft and 51 (8,31%) with Dacron. Extensive and detailed information regarding published data are shown in the Table 4.

6. Conclusion

When it comes to carotid stenosis, EA is the method of choice in majority of patients. Small subgroup of patients had extensive carotid atherosclerotic disease that involves common or internal carotid artery in a segment longer than 4cm. In these situations modification of surgical procedure is necessary since EA might be jeopardized. Optimal scenario would be to assess extension of atherosclerotic process preoperatively through ultrasonography or MSCT angiography or intraoperatively during dissection of carotid arteries. In case of extensive atherosclerotic process, decision to perform carotid graft replacement without any attempt of EA could simplify procedure, shorten cross clamping time and avoid technical and thromboembolic complications. Conduit choice is the matter of operating surgeon. Upon clamping and resecting diseased segment, suturing distal anastomosis first is recommendable in order to provide easier manipulation and better visualization of anastomotic line. Next step is suturing the proximal anastomosis then flushing and finally carotid declamping. Reimplantation of external carotid artery is not mandatory and the decision should be made as the preference of the surgeon. Efforts to perform EA even in case of extensive disease could be effective especially in experienced hands, however in case of any doubts in wall quality or end of the plaque zone, graft replacement should be performed before flow restoration in order to prevent fatal complications that this procedure carries.

There is not enough evidence to provide any accurate criteria for usage of carotid graft replacement instead of endarterectomy. This chapter showed results, experience and technical details of a single high volume center and presented not so reach published material. Decision to perform graft replacement should be made individually according to anatomy and morphology of carotid disease. Wide surgical experience affords expertise and improves individual decision making.

Author details

Igor Koncar, Nikola Ilic, Marko Dragas, Miroslav Markovic, Dusan Kostic and Lazar Davidovic
Clinic for Vascular and Endovascular Surgery, Serbian Clinical Centre, Serbia
Medical Faculty, University of Belgrade, Serbia

Igor Banzic
Clinic for Vascular and Endovascular Surgery, Serbian Clinical Centre, Serbia

Acknowledgments

Authors would like to thank to Katarina Kaplarski for providing illustrations of the procedure.

Presented study is a part of a scientific research project (Grant OI175008) supported by the Ministry of Education and Science of the Republic of Serbia.

7. References

[1] Chiari H: Ueber Verhalten Teilungswinkels der Carotis communis bei der Endarteritis chronica deformans. Verh Dtsch Pathol Ges 1905; 9:326-330.

[2] Moniz E, Lima A, de Lacerda R: Hemiplegies par thrombose de la carotide interne.Presse Med 1937; 45:977-980.

[3] Carrea R, Molins M, Murphy G: Surgical treatment of spontaneous thrombosis of the internal carotid artery in the neck: carotid-carotideal anastomosis.Report of a case.Acta Neurol Latinoamer 1955; 1:71-78.

[4] Eastcott HHG, Pickering GW, Rob CG: Reconstruction of internal carotid artery in a patient with intermittent attacks of hemiplegia. Lancet 1954; 2:994-996.

[5] Debakey ME: Successful carotid endarterectomy for cerebrovascular insufficiency: nineteen year follow-up. JAMA 1975; 233:1083-1085.

[6] Rowe WF. An early successful carotid endarterectomy, not previously reported. Paper presented at the Annual Meeting of the Southern California Vascular Surgical Society, September 18th, 1993, Coronado, CA

[7] Cooley DA, Al-Naaman YD, Carton CA: Surgical treatment of arteriosclerotic occlusion of the common carotid artery.J Neurosurg 1956; 13:500-506

[8] North American Symptomatic Carotid Endarterectomy Trial Collaborators: Beneficial effect of carotid endarterectomy in symptomatic patients with high-grade carotid stenosis. N Engl J Med 1991; 325:445-453.

[9] North American Symptomatic Carotid Endarterectomy Trial Collaborators: Benefit of carotid endarterectomy in patients with symptomatic moderate or severe stenosis. N Engl J Med 1998; 339:1415-1425.

[10] European Carotid Surgery Trialists' Collaborative Group: MRC European Carotid Surgery Trial: interim results for patients with severe (70-99%) or mild (0-29%) carotid stenosis. Lancet 1991; 337:1235-1243.

[11] Executive Committee of the Asymptomatic Carotid Atherosclerosis Study: Endarterectomy for asymptomatic carotid artery stenosis. JAMA 1995; 273:1421-1428.

[12] ACST Collaborators Group: The International Asymptomatic Carotid Surgery Trial (ACST). Lancet 2004; 363:1491-1502.

[13] Alison Halliday, Michael Harrison, Elizabeth Hayter, Xiangling Kong, Averil Mansfield, Joanne Marro, Hongchao Pan, Richard Peto, John Potter, Kazem Rahimi, Angela Rau, Stephen Robertson, Jonathan Streifler, Dafydd Thomas, on behalf of the Asymptomatic Carotid Surgery Trial (ACST) Collaborative Group*10-year stroke

prevention after successful carotid endarterectomy for asymptomatic stenosis (ACST-1): a multicentre randomised trial. Lancet 2010; 376: 1074–84

[14] LeFevre H: Sur un cas de plaie du bulbe carotidien per balle, traitee par la ligature de la carotid primitive, et l'anastomose bout et bout de la carotid externe avec la carotid interne. Bull Mem Soc Chir 1918; 44:923-928.

[15] Dimitza A: Aneurysms of the carotid arteries. Report of 2 cases. Angiology 1956; 7:218-227.

[16] Beall Jr AC, Crawford ES, Cooley DA, DeBakey ME: Extracranial aneurysms of the carotid artery. Report of seven cases. Postgrad Med 1962; 32:93-102.

[17] Vaughan GD, Mattox KL, Feliciano DV, Beall AC Jr, DeBakey ME. Surgical experience with expanded polytetrafluoroethylene (ePTFE) as a replacement graft for traumatized vessels. J Trauma 1979;19:403-98.

[18] Denman FR, Ehni G, Duty WS. Insidious thrombotic oclusion of cervical carotid arteries, treated by arterial graft; a case report. Surgery 1955, 38 (3): 569-77.

[19] Doyle EJ, Javid H, Lin PM. Partial internal carotid artery occlusion treated by primary resection and vein graft; report of a case. Jneurosurg 1956, 13 (6): 650-5.

[20] Dos Santos JC: Sur la desobstion des thromboses arterielles anciennes. Mem Acad Chir 1947; 73:409.

[21] Wylie EJ, Kerr E, Davies O: Experimental and clinical experiences with the use of fascia lata applied as a graft about major arteries after thromboendarterectomy and aneurysmorrhaphy. Surg Gynecol Obstet 1951; 93:257.

[22] Van der Akker PJ, van Schilfaarde R: Long-term results of prosthetic and non-prosthetic reconstruction for obstructive aorto-iliac disease. Eur J Vasc Surg 1992; 6:53.

[23] Stoney RJ, Reilly LM: Endarterectomy for aortoiliac occlusive disease. In: Ernst CB, Stanley JC, ed. Current Therapy in Vascular Therapy, Philadelphia: BC Decker; 1987:157.

[24] Inahara T: Evaluation of endarterectomy for aortoiliac and aortoilio-femoral occlusive disease. Arch Surg 1975; 110:1458.

[25] Brewster DC, Darling RC: Optimal methods of aortoiliac reconstruction. Surgery 1978; 84:739.

[26] Darling RC, Paty PS, Shah DM, Chang BB, Leather RP. Eversion endarterectomy of the internal carotid artery: technique and results in 449 procedures. Surgery. 1996;120(4):635–639.

[27] Cao PG, de Rango P, Zannetti S, Giordano G, Ricci S, Celani MG. Eversion versus conventional carotid endarterectomy for preventing stroke. Cochrane Database Syst Rev 2001;(1). CD001921

[28] Markovic DM, Davidovic LB, Cvetkovic DD, Maksimovic ZV,Markovic DZ, Jadranin DB. Single-center prospective, randomized analysis of conventional and eversion carotid endarterectomy. J Cardiovasc Surg (Torino) 2008;49(5):619-25.

[29] Ballotta E, Da Giau G, Saladini M, Abbruzzese E, Renon L, Toniato A. Carotid endarterectomy with patch closure versus carotid eversion endarterectomy and reimplantation: a prospective randomized study. Surgery 1999;125(3):271-9

[30] Kieny R, Hirsch D, Seiller C, Thiranos JC, Petit H. Does carotid eversion endarterectomy and reimplantation reduce the risk of restenosis? Ann Vasc Surg 1993;7(5):407-13

[31] Raithel D. Carotid eversion endarterectomy: a better technique than the standard operation? Cardiovasc Surg 1997;5(5):471-2.

[32] Liapis CD, Bell PR, Mikhailidis D, Sivenius J, Nicolaides A, Fernandes e Fernandes J, et al. ESVS guidelines. Invasive treatment for carotid stenosis: indications, techniques. Eur J Vasc Endovasc Surg 2009;37(4 Suppl):1-19

[33] C.D. Mann, M. McCarthy, A. Nasim, M. Bown, M. Dennis, R. Sayers, N. London, A.R. Naylor. Management and Outcome of Prosthetic Patch Infection after Carotid Endarterectomy: A Single-centre Series and Systematic Review of the Literature Eur J Vasc Endovasc Surg 44 (2012) 20-26

[34] C. Liapis, W.C. Mackey, B. Perler, P. Cao Comparison of SVS and ESVS Carotid Disease Management Guidelines Eur J Vasc Endovasc Surg (2009) 38, 243-245

[35] A History of Vascular Surgery SECOND EDITION, Steven G. Friedman, Blackwell Publishing, Inc, 2005

[36] Berguer R, Kieffer E. (1992): Surgery of the Arteries to the Head, Springer-Verlag, New York, Berlin, Heidelberg, 74 -206.

[37] Vaughan GD, Mattox KL, Feliciano DV, Beall AC Jr, DeBakey ME.Surgical experience with expanded polytetrafluoroethylene (ePTFE) as a replacement graft for traumatized vessels. J Trauma 1979;19:403-98.

[38] Cormier F, Laurian C, Gigou F, Fichelle JM, Bokobza B. Polytetrafluoroethylene bypass for revascularization of the atherosclerotic internal carotid artery: late results Annals Of Vascular Surgery , 1987 Dec;1(5):564-71

[39] Christophe Camiade, Amer Maher, Jean-Baptiste Ricco, Jerome Roumy, Guillaume Febrer, Christophe Marchand, Jean-Philippe Neau. Carotid bypass with polytetrafluoroethylene grafts: A study of 110 consecutive patients. J Vasc Surg 2003;38:1031-8.

[40] Sise MJ, Ivy ME, Malanche R, Ranbarger KR. Polytetrafluoroethylene interposition grafts for carotid reconstruction. J Vasc Surg 1992;16:601-8.

[41] Becquemin JP, Cavillon A, Brunel M, Desgranges P, Melliere D. Polytetrafluorethylene grafts for carotid repair. Cardiovasc Surg 1996;4:740-5.

[42] Henry C. Veldeniz, Rhea Kinser, George Neil Yates. Carotid graft replacement: A durable option J Vasc Surg 2005;42:220-6.

[43] Branchereau A, Pietri P, Magnan PE, Rosset E. Saphenous vein bypass: an alternative to internal carotid reconstruction. Eur J Vasc Endovasc Surg 1996;12:26-30.

[44] Voirin L, Magne JL, Farah I, Sessa C, Chichignoud B, Guidicelli H. Carotid revascularizations by venous grafting: long-term results. Chirurgie (Paris) 1997;122:346-50.

[45] Fabiani JN, Julia P, Chemla E, Birnbaum PL, Chardigny C, D'Attellis N, et al. Is the incidence of recurrent carotid artery stenosis influenced by the choice of the surgical technique: carotid endarterectomy versus saphenous vein bypass. J Vasc Surg 1994;20:821-5.

[46] C. Lauder, A. Kelly, M. M. Thompson, N. J. M. London, P. R. F. Bell, A. R. Naylor. Early and late outcome after carotid artery bypass grafting with saphenous vein J Vasc Surg 2003;38:1025-30.

[47] Amir H Dorafshar, Todd D Reil, Samuel S Ahn, William J Quinones-Baldrich, Wesley S Moore Interposition Grafts for Difficult Carotid Artery Reconstruction: A 17-Year Experience Ann Vasc Surg. 2007 Dec 11; : 18082917 (P,S,E,B,D).

[48] Radak D, Davidovic L, Tanaskovic S, Koncar I, Babic S, Kostic D, Ilijevski N. Surgical treatment of carotid restenosis after eversion endarterectomy-serbian bicentric prospective study. Ann Vasc Surg. 2012 Aug;26(6):783-9.

[49] Radak D, Davidović L, Vukobratov V, Ilijevski N, Kostić D, Maksimović Z, Vucurević G, Cvetkovic S, Avramov S. Carotid artery aneurysms: Serbian Multicentric Study. Ann Vasc Surg. 2007 Jan;21(1):23-9.

Chapter 2

Simultaneous Hybrid Revascularization by Carotid Stenting and Coronary Artery Bypass Grafting – The SHARP Study

Luigi Chiariello, Paolo Nardi and Francesco Versaci

Additional information is available at the end of the chapter

1. Introduction

Significant atherosclerotic disease affecting also the carotid artery system is encountered in a substantial number of patients undergoing coronary artery bypass grafting (CABG) [1]. The optimal surgical management to prevent stroke and cardiac events in this subset of patients remains unclear [2-5]. Among patients undergoing carotid endoarterectomy (CEA) procedure in the Veterans Affair Cooperative Study and in the Asymptomatic Carotid Atherosclerosis Study, respectively 20% and 49% of deaths were related to cardiac causes [4]. Similarly, the incidence of perioperative stroke in patients undergoing CABG is high in those affected by concomitant significant carotid disease [2-4]. The combined surgical approach is associated with an increased risk for mortality and morbidity [5]. In the staged surgical approach which addresses the carotid artery lesion with carotid endoarterectomy first, followed several days to several weeks by CABG, incidence of perioperative stroke during CABG is reduced .However, the risk of myocardial infarction (MI) during the CEA procedure and in the period preceding CABG remains high (6%) [6]. Carotid artery stenting (CAS) using cerebral protection devices is rapidly evolving as an alternative to carotid endoarterectomy [7], mainly for patients with severe carotid artery stenosis at high surgical risk [8], such as patients with coronary artery disease. A staged CAS-CABG approach has been recently proposed, but the need of a dual anti-platelet aggregation therapy lasting 3-4 weeks after stenting may represent a limitation for CABG [9].

2. Clinical experience

In our Institution in 2005 we introduced a new therapeutic strategy consisting of a simultaneous hybrid revascularization by CAS, immediately followed by CABG and cases have been colleted in the SHARP study ("Simultaneous hybrid revascularization by carotid artery stenting and coronary artery bypass grafting") (Figure 1).

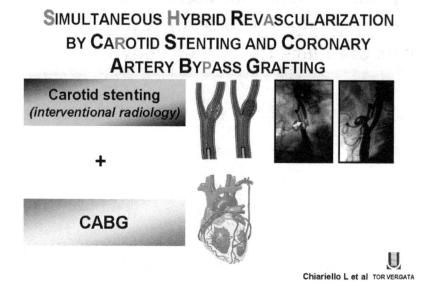

SIMULTANEOUS HYBRID REVASCULARIZATION BY CAROTID STENTING AND CORONARY ARTERY BYPASS GRAFTING

Carotid stenting
(interventional radiology)

+

CABG

Chiariello L et al TOR VERGATA

Figure 1.

As compared to the combined or staged surgical strategy currently adopted, the new hybrid approach CAS-CABG can reduce the incidence of serious perioperative adverse events and minimize surgical trauma. Surgical time and surgical trauma are shorter and less extensive as compared to combined CEA and CABG. Risk of MI is expected to be reduced, by shortening the interval between the two procedures [10, 11].

Eligible criteria for the enrolment: 1) concomitant critical carotid and coronary disease with coronary arteries suitable for CABG; 2) EuroSCORE ≥5; 3) a carotid artery stenosis ≥50% in the symptomatic disease or ≥80% in asymptomatic disease, as determined by the North American Symptomatic Carotid Endarterectomy Trial (NASCET) criteria [2]. The presence of carotid artery stenosis was evidenced by eco duplex scanning, then confirmed by catheter angiography and either magnetic resonance angiography or computed tomography (CT) scan angiography. A CT scan with or without angiographic dye, depending on preprocedural serum levels of creatinine, was performed in all patients to provide the maximum information regarding the aortic arch, the extent of aortic disease and the brain. In case of bilateral carotid artery stenosis the choice of the carotid artery to treat was made according to clinical criteria or to the severity and morphology of plaque in case of asymptomatic patients. In a very few instances of bilateral subocclusive carotid stenosis, successful bilateral CAS has been performed, immediately followed by CABG.

CAS procedures were performed under local anaesthesia through a percutaneous transfemoral access with the use of stents and protection devices. An introducer sheath was positioned in the femoral artery, and heparin (1 mg /kg) was administered intra-arterially as a bolus. Then a guiding catheter was placed in the common carotid artery, proximally to the bifurcation. A distal filter protection was used in all patients. At the end of the procedure, patients were transferred directly to the operating room; CABG procedure was performed by means of normothermic cardiopulmonary bypass in the majority patients; in few cases off-pump CABG procedure was performed according with the choice of surgeon and comorbidity of patient.

2.1. Periprocedural pharmacological protocol

Aspirin 100 mg daily was started at least 2 days before CAS and daily after combined procedure was performed. Heparin was administered 1 mg /Kg as a bolus intra-arterially immediately before the stent implantation procedure and in the operating room before the cardiopulmonary bypass 2 mg/Kg as a bolus. Activated clotting time was checked every 30 minutes and was constantly maintained $\geq$ 250 sec. until the CABG procedure and $\geq$480 seconds until the end of the cardiopulmonary bypass. Tranexamic acid 2 g in bolus was administered as an antifibrinolytic agent over 20 minutes before sternotomy and then as endovenous infusion (0.5 g/h) until the patient was admitted to the postoperative intensive care unit in most of cases. Clopidogrel, 300 mg as a loading dose, followed by 75 mg per day for 1 month was started in the intensive care unit via a nasogastric tube 6 hours after the end of CABG surgery, providing that surgical bleeding from the thoracic drains had either stopped, or when it was less than 50 mL/hr for 3 consecutive hours from the sixth postoperative hour on (Figure 2).

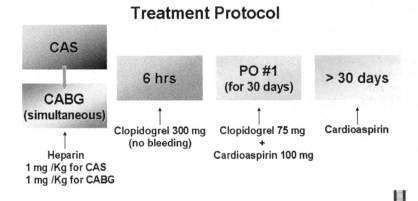

Figure 2.

The primary end points analyzed were the incidence of stroke, MI or death at 30 days after CAS-CABG and at a mid-term follow-up.

2.2. In-hospital and follow-up results

One-hundred and forty eight consecutive patients between January 2005 and November 2011 underwent CAS-CABG treatment. Mean age of patients was 68±8 years, means EuroSCORE 8.6±2.5; 22 patients (14.8%) were affected by symptomatic carotid disease; 67 (45%) had bilateral carotid stenosis. Left internal mammary artery was used as graft to the left anterior descending artery in all patients, bilateral mammary artery in 20 cases (13.5%). (Table 1).

Variable	Value
Number of patients	148
Age - years *	68 ± 8
Male - n. † (%)	118 (79)
CCS pre-op - mean *	2.7 ± 1
CCS class III/IV ‡ - n. (%)	93 (63)
Instable Angina- n. (%)	34 (23)
NYHA – mean *	2.2 ± 1
Bilateral carotid stenosis- n. (%)	67 (45)
Previous Stroke o TIA - n. (%)	22 (14,8)
Surgical Risk**	8.6 ± 2.5
Doppler velocity of internal carotid artery. - mean *	325 ± 40 cm/sec

* ± DS
† n. = number
‡ Following classification of Canadian Cardiovascular Society (CCS).
§ Sierum creatinin concentration >1,5 mg/dl and clearence of creatinin <50 ml/min.
** Surgical Risk as EuroSCORE I (Eur J Cardiothor Surg 1999; 15:816-823).
MI= miocardial infarction; LVEF =Left ventrical ejection fraction.

Table 1. Preoperative details of patients.

Clinical major outcomes at 48 months are reported in Table 2

Operative mortality	1.3%
Periprocedural Stroke	1.3%
Perioperative MI	0
Re-exploration for bleeding	2.0%
Stroke, MI or death within 48 months	6.1%

MI = myocardial infarction

Table 2. Incidence of Clinical Events up to 48 months

In the first one hundred patients we report a mean follow-up of 40±25 months, 97% complete. In these patients we found at the end of follow-up 9 deaths whit a cumulative survival rate of 89%; furthermore we observed a very low mortality rate for cardiac late death (97±2%) and an high rate of freedom from fatal stroke (we registered just one case of fatal stroke during follow-up) (98±2%), MI (96±3%), and cerebrovascular events (90±6%). (Figure 3-6)

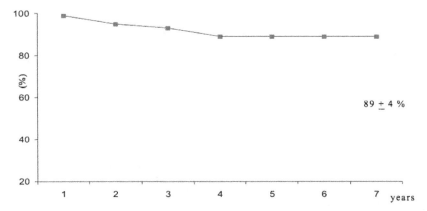

Figure 3. Survival rate at follow-up

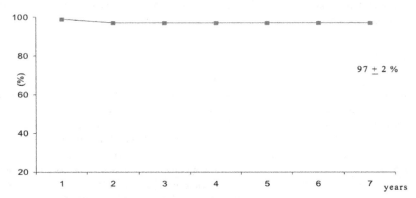

Figure 4. Kaplan Meier: Freedom from cardiac late death.

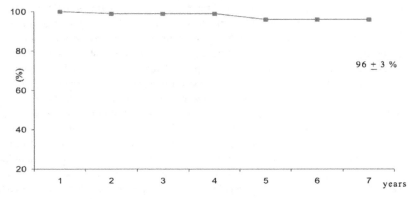

Figure 5. Kaplan Meier: Freedom from miocardial infarction.

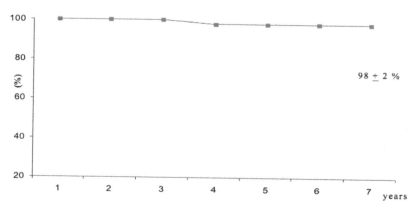

Figure 6. Kaplan Meier: freedom from fatal stroke.

Internal carotid artery systolic blood flow during follow-up, showed significant improvement as compared to preoperative mean value. (67±10 cm/sec vs. 325±40 cm/sec, $P < .001$).

3. Comments

Neurological complications are relatively common after CABG, especially in high-risk patients. Carotid artery disease is significantly associated with a type I adverse neurological outcome (i.e., death due to stroke or hypoxic encephalopathy, nonfatal stroke, TIA, stupor, or coma at the time of discharge). Significant carotid artery stenoses are associated with up to 30% of early postoperative strokes following CABG. Preventing stroke and cardiovascular events after CABG is an important and complex issue. Concomitant carotid artery disease might be a major factor contributing to the occurrence of postoperative stroke. Moreover, carotid artery disease might be a marker of diffuse atherosclerosis, affecting also aortic arch, arch vessels, and intracranial vessels. In this high risk population, a simplified operative management like hybrid revascularization by CAS and CABG can minimize the negative impact of diffuse atherosclerotic disease. In fact, our findings indicate that, in patients with combined carotid artery disease and coronary artery disease, the proposed hybrid approach is a feasible therapeutic option with good immediate and short-term clinical results. The recently reported incidence of perioperative stroke and mortality following CEA and CABG is not negligible, ranging between 8.3% to 10.3% [12]. According to these results, in a previous series of 100 consecutive patients undergoing combined surgical revascularization at our Institution between 1991 and 2002, the 30-day mortality and stroke rate was 10% and 1.1%, respectively, with a mortality rate of 14.5% when the standard EuroSCORE was ≥ 6, and 3.4% when it was lower than 6. These high-risk patients could be treated by an alternative strategy such as the hybrid approach proposed in this study. As compared with combined surgical revascularization, the hybrid strategy requires a shorter surgical time and less extensive surgical trauma, thus reducing cofactors known to increase morbidity and mortality. In particular, in high-risk patients for CEA, mainly due to severe CAD, the SAPPHIRE (Stenting and Angioplasty with Protection in Patients at High

Risk for Endarterectomy) trial showed that CAS was safer than carotid endarterectomy, because it had a lower postprocedural risk of myocardial infarction at 30 days as compared with surgery. This is likely to be the case mainly in patients with elevated surgical risk, such as the patients involved in the SHARP study. In particular, when the standard EuroSCORE is 8, as it is in our study, the surgical mortality rate might be greater than 10-12%. In this high-risk subset of patients, specific surgical complications are also increased up to 55% [13]. When both internal carotid arteries have significant stenosis, the risk of stroke after cardiac surgery is particularly high (25%). With the percutaneous hybrid approach, in our study the stroke rate was only 1.3%, considering that 45% of our patients had bilateral internal carotid artery disease. Potential adjunctive advantage of the simultaneous hybrid approach as compared with a combined surgical approach is that during the CAS procedure the patient is awake and the neurological outcome will be known instantly rather than after the patient emerges from general anaesthesia. Another most important finding of our study was the absence of periprocedural rate of MI. By observing the proposed protocol, the risk of MI, especially during carotid surgery or in the time elapsing between the two procedures (CEA or CAS and CABG after 3-4 weeks from carotid procedure), is virtually eliminated. In the two-stage procedure, the rate of MI when the patient is waiting for CABG after carotid artery procedure is about 5-6%. Finally our study also demonstrated safety of the pharmacological protocol and the timing of antiplatelet administration proposed: the bleeding rate after surgical intervention was low.

The proposed hybrid approach conferred an operative mortality rate comparable to that of isolated CABG.

In conclusions, the new hybrid approach is aiming to reduce risk of myocardial infarction, of bleeding after CABG and risk of death and major cerebrovascular complications. Reduced mortality and morbidity are expected to reduce also in-hospital stay and costs. Therefore, in patients with combined carotid artery and coronary artery disease at higher surgical risk, the proposed hybrid approach seems to be a possible, advantageous and safe alternative therapeutic strategy.

At a mid-term period, a high rate of event-free survival and freedom from cerebrovascular events can be expected.

Author details

Luigi Chiariello*, Paolo Nardi and Francesco Versaci
Cardiac Surgery Unit, Fondazione Policlinico Università Tor Vergata, Rome, Italy

4. References

[1] Alboyans V, Lacroix P. Indications for carotid screening in patients with carotid artery disease. Presse Med 2009;38(6):977-86

---

* Corresponding Author

[2] Mackey WC, O'Donnell TF, Callow AD. Cardiac risk in patients undergoing carotid endoarterectomy: impact on perioperative and long-term mortality. J Vasc Surg 1990;11:226-33.

[3] North American Symptomatic Carotid Endarterectomy Trial Collaborators. Beneficial effect of carotid endoarterectomy in symptomatic patients with high-grade of carotid stenosis. N Engl J Med 1991;325:445-53.

[4] European Carotid Surgery Trialist' Collaborative Group. MRC European Carotid Surgical Trial: interim results for symptomatic patients with severe (70-99%) or with mild (0-29%) carotid stenosis. Lancet 1991;337:1235-43.

[5] Executive committee for the asymptomatic carotid atherosclerosis study: Endarterectomy for Asymptomatic Carotid Atherosclerosis Study. JAMA 1995;273:1421-8.

[6] Naylor AR, Cuffe RL, Rothwell PM, Bell PR. A systematic review of outcomes following staged and synchronous carotid endarterectomy and coronary artery bypass. Eur J Vasc Endovasc Surg 2003;25(5):380-9.

[7] Brott TG, Hobson RW 2nd, Howard G at al. Stenting versus endarterectomy for treatment of carotid artery stenosis. N Engl J Med 2010;363(1):11-23.

[8] Gum HS, Yadav JS, Fayad P et al. Long term results of carotid stenting versus endarterectomy in high risk patients. N Engl J Med 2008;358(15):1572-9.

[9] Lopes DK, Mericle RA, Lanzino G et al. Stent placement for the treatment of occlusive atherosclerotic carotid artery disease in patients with concomitant coronary artery disease. J Neurosurg 2002; 96(3): 490-6.

[10] Yadav JS, Wholey MH, Kuntz RE, Fayad P, Katzen BT, Mishkel GJ, Bajwa TK, Whitlow P, Strickman NE, Jaff MR, Popma JJ, Snead DB, Cutlip DE, Firth BG, Ouriel K; Stenting and Angioplasty with Protection in Patients at High Risk for Endarterectomy Investigators. Protected carotid-artery stenting versus endarterectomy in high-risk patients. N Engl J Med 2004;351:1493-501.

[11] Chiariello L, Tomai F, Zeitani J, Versaci F. Simultaneous hybrid revascularization by carotid stenting and coronary artery bypass grafting. Ann Thorac Surg 2006;81:1833-5.

[12] Versaci F, Del Giudice C, Scafuri A, Zeitani J, Gandini R, Nardi P, Salvati A, Pampana E, Sebastiano F, Romagnoli A, Simonetti G, Chiariello L. Sequential hybrid carotid and coronary artery revascularization: immediate and mid-term results. Ann Thorac Surg 2007;84:1508-14.

[13] Hertze NR, Mascha EJ. A personal experience with coronary artery bypass grafting, carotid patching, and other factors influencing the outcome of carotid endarterectomy. J Vasc Surg 2006;43:959-68.

[14] Fukuda M, Takagi Y. Application of preoperative risk severity evaluation system (EuroSCORE, European system for cardiac operative risk evaluation) for cardiac operative patients). Masui 2004;53:1149-54.

Perioperative Care

Chapter 3

Current Management of Vascular Infections

Kiriakos Ktenidis and Argyrios Giannopoulos

Additional information is available at the end of the chapter

1. Introduction

Technical advances in Vascular Surgery have led to an increased use of prostheses (grafts, patches, stents, stent grafts etc.) and improved results for the patient. Despite routine antibiotic prophylaxis, infection, although rare, remains a serious complication, with catastrophic consequences. Vascular infections are divided into 3 groups according to Szilagyi (Table 1.), depending on the extent of the inflammation: the superficial, the deep and the mixed type.[1] Samson (Table 1.), as well as Karl and Storck (Table 1.) , have modified the widely used classification system of Szilagyi.[1-3] While the superficial type is restricted to the skin and subcutaneous tissue, the deep infection involves the vessels or a prosthetic graft. The mixed type of vascular infection is the combination of the above types affects all the tissue layers and can produce trauma disruption. Vascular infections can be classified by appearance time into: a) early (<4 weeks after graft implantation) and b) late (>4 weeks). Samson's and Karl's modifications take into consideration further clinical parameters, which define the treatment (Table 2.). [2,3] When infection involves a graft anastomosis or the suture line of a patch, there is high risk of vessel rupture, septic hemorrhage or pseudoaneurysm formation. [4-6] Other serious complications are septic thrombosis, endocarditis, etc. [7] In severe cases, treatment can be problematic and mortality remains high, despite the use of antibiotics and surgical treatment. Keys to successful outcome include early and accurate diagnosis, identification of the infecting organism, and extent of graft infection, administration of culture-specific antibiotic therapy, and excision or replacement of the infected graft.

2. Epidemiology

The reported incidence of infection involving vascular prosthesis varies, occurring after 0.2% to 5% of vascular procedures . [4] The long - term incidence is possibly higher than that reported, since some graft infections (e.g. aortic graft infections) develop several years after implantation . [8]

Groups	Szilagyi	Samson	Karl-Storck
I	infection involves only the dermis	infections extend no deeper than the dermis	Superficial infection without involvement of the graft
II	infection extends into the subcutaneous tissue but does not invade the arterial implant	infections involve subcutaneous tissues but do not come into grossly observable direct contact with the graft	Partial graft infection without involvement of the anastomosis
III	the arterial implant proper is involved in the infection	infections involve the body of the graft but not at an anastomosis	involvement of the anastomosis and suture line
IV		infections surround an exposed anastomosis but bacteremia or anastomotic bleeding has not occurred	Wound disruption and complete exposure of the graft/patch
V		infections involve a graft-to-artery anastomosis and are associated with septicemia and/or bleeding at the time of presentation	All the above groups with concomitant septic bleeding/pseudoaneurysm
VI			All the above groups with graft thrombosis or septic emboli

Table 1. Classification of vascular graft infections

Grade	Clinical findings	Recommendation
Szilagyi I, Samson I	Infection involves only cutis	Conservative treatment
Szilagyi II, Samson II, Karl I	Cutis/subcutis infection without graft involvement	a) graft preservation combined with VAC b) graft excision
Szilagyi III, Samson III, Karl II	Deep graft infection without involvement of anastomosis or suture line	a) graft preservation combined with VAC b) graft excision
Szilagyi III, Samson IV, Karl III-IV	Deep graft infection with involvement of anastomosis or suture line	a) graft excision b) graft preservation combined with VAC
Szilagyi III, Samson V, Karl V-VI	Deep graft infection associated with complications (bleeding, thrombosis, suture aneurysm)	graft excision

Table 2. Therapeutic recommendations depending on the infection grade

Incidence of vascular infections is influenced by patient's general condition, the type of the procedure, the coexistence of other simultaneous inflammation sites, the type of prophylactic antibiotics given perioperatively and by prolonged operative time and hospital stay . [9-13] Infections are much more frequent in the groins (60% of cases), in grafts placed in a subcutaneous tunnel and after emergency cases (e.g. acute arterial ischemia). Infection can also develop after percutaneous stent angioplasty but in low rates (0.5%). [14,15]

Early graft infections usually affect extracavitary grafts, while majority of late infections involve cavitary (i.e., aortic) grafts. [16]

3. Pathogenesis

Exposure of vascular grafts to bacteria, irrespective of source, may result in colonization and subsequent infection. Microorganisms can result in clinical infection most commonly, perioperatively, during surgical implantation or through the surgical wound. The most common mechanisms of infection are: break of aseptic techniques in the operating room and contact of the graft with patient's endogenous flora harboured in lymphatics rupturing intraoperatively, sweat glands or mucosas. Intraoperative injury of gastrointestinal or genitourinary tract, diseased arterial wall, healing problems of surgical wound and reoperations can result in graft infection. [4]

Bacterial contamination of the prosthesis via a hematogenous route is rare, though urinary tract infections, infected intravascular catheters, pneumonia or other remote tissue infections (e.g. infected foot ulcer) increase the risk of graft infection. Bacteremia can result in graft infection, years after the implantation, especially in elderly patients with altered immune status.

Moreover, erosion of a prosthetic graft through the skin or into the gastrointestinal or genitourinary tract can lead to an infection. GEE/GEF can develop due to pulsatile pressure transmitted via an aortic graft to the overlying adherent bowel, usually the third part of the duodenum. This can be prevented by coverage of the graft by adjacent omentum at the end of the procedure. A graft-cutaneous fistula by erosion through intact skin is most commonly the result of a low-grade infection caused by S. epidermidis.

Finally, grafts can get contaminated by a contiguous infectious process as a result of an adjacent infection (e.g. diverticulitis, infected lymphocele).

Predisposing factors for vascular infection are the use of prosthetic grafts, procedures in the groins, local or systemic septic conditions, while the predicting factors are patient's immune status, graft's characteristics, prolonged hospital stay , bacterial virulence or resistance to antibiotics. Additionally, reoperations, long or emergency procedures, faulty sterile surgical technique, postoperative complications (such as hematoma, graft thrombosis) and concomitant urological or biliary and colon operations contribute to increased rates of vascular infections. [17]

4. Bacteriology

Staphylococci (*Staphylococcus aureus* and coagulase negative staphylococci) account for more than 75% of vascular device-related infections. In fact, *S. aureus* is the most prevalent pathogen. Graft infections due to *S. epidermidis* or gram-negative bacteria have increased in frequency. Less frequently, microorganisms of the skin flora, such as streptococci and *Propionibacterium acnes*, are isolated.

Gram-negative bacteria such as *Pseudomonas, E. coli, Klebsiella, Enterobacter,* and *Proteus* species are particularly virulent, followed by high rates of anastomotic disruption. This can be explained by their ability to produce toxins, such as elastase and alkaline protease, which can decompose the arterial wall. [18,19]

MRSA (Methicillin-resistant *S. aureus)* vascular infections present with increased incidence. [20] Fungal infections are rare and develop usually in immunosuppressed patients.

Early infections are usually caused by especially virulent microorganisms, such as S. aureus, Streptococcus faecalis, E. coli, Pneumococcus, Klebsiella and Proteus. Late infections are the result of low-virulence microorganisms such as S. Epidermidis.

5. Clinical manifestations

Clinical manifestations vary according to the localization of the vessel that is involved. Graft infections in limbs (e.g. femoropopliteal graft) present with edema, cellulitis or with a pulsatile mass, in case anastomotic rupture and pseudoaneurysm formation. According to Szilagyi, vascular infections can be classified by relationship to postoperative wound infection. Graft contamination in the abdominal (Table 3.) or thoracic cavity, usually presents with systematic sepsis, aortoenteric, and aortobrochial or aortooesophageal fistula. Symptoms in early infections can be fever, leukocytosis and perigraft purulence.

Patients with aortic grafts and gastrointestinal bleeding should be investigated for GEE. [21,22] Bacteremia develops in advanced graft infections. Graft infection due to *S. epidermidis* typically presents months to years after graft implantation with anastomotic aneurysm, graft-cutaneous sinus tract or perigraft cavity with fluid. Vascular Surgeon should, also, look for other sources of infection, (e.g. feet or urinary infections).

6. Diagnosis

6.1. Laboratory testing

Early diagnosis is crucial for treatment and for prevention of septic complications that can threaten the affected limb or even patient's life. It is based on physical examination and imaging modalities. Blood tests results are non-specific for vascular infection, with low diagnostic value. Elevated WBC count with left shifted differential, increased erythrocyte sedimentation rate or high levels of CRP can be found during the acute phase. Blood cultures are rarely positive (<5%) but such findings, in addition with high fever, are markers of advanced infection and sepsis. In these cases, early hospital admission and treatment are essential. Laboratory tests should include cultures from other sites of infection and stool guaiac, in case GEE is suspected.

Type of graft infection	Time from implantation	Microorganisms
Periprosthetic infection	Early (< 4 mo)	Staphylococcus aureus, Streptococcus, Escherichia Coli, Pseudomonas
	Late (> 4 mo)	Staphylococcus epidermidis
Entero-paraprosthetic	Late	Escherichia coli, Enterococcus, Bacteroides infection
Aorto-enteric fistula	Early	Escherichia coli, Staphylococcus aureus
	Late	Escherichia coli, Klebsiella, Staphylococcus epidermidis

Table 3. Classification of aortic graft infection (Bandyk 1991)

6.2. Vascular imaging

Vascular imaging is of crucial significance in the diagnosis and treatment planning of vascular infections. Imaging modalities that are useful for diagnosis are ultrasonography, CT Angiography, MR Angiography, endoscopy or functional radionuclide imaging (indium 111-labelled leukocytes). The combination of anatomic and functional vascular imaging techniques shows high sensitivity (80% to 100%) and specificity (50% to 90%) in identification of infection.

Plain radiographs are of limited value, providing information only in the case of prosthesis misplacement or dislocation.

Color duplex scanning is a readily available imaging technique, reliable for diagnosis of perigraft fluid collection, which can be differentiated from anastomotic pseudoaneurysms, especially in extracavitary infections. Imaging of abdominal cavity or aortic grafts is not accurate in obese patients. Graft patency can be easily examined.

Contrast-enhanced CT is the preferred imaging technique for abdominal or thoracic aorta graft infections. Signs of abnormal fluid or gas collections around the prosthesis (beyond 2-3 months of implantation) or false aneurysm formation are suggestive of infection. Loss of normal retroperitoneal tissue planes or vertebral osteomyelitis in a patient with an aortic graft indicates a vascular infection. CT-guided aspiration is being increasingly used to differentiate perigraft abcesses from seromas.

MRA is an alternative modality to CTA, with equal specificity or sensitivity. It can also differentiate perigraft fluid from adjacent fibrosis. Gadolinium is less nephrotoxic in patients with renal insufficiency. However, it is contraindicated in patients with electrophysiological devices. The presence of metallic materials may cause artefacts that compromise image quality.

The use of arteriography is useful in the identification of anastomotic aneurysms or other graft complications (e.g. graft rupture) and for the evaluation of the vascular tree before revascularization planning. It should be a routine examination in hemodynamically stable patients with graft infection unless CT or MRI scans give the above type of information.

Functional White Blood Cell Scanning is indicated in special cases. 99mTc-labelled white blood cells, 111In or gallium scintigrams are most commonly used along with MRI and CT to define the extent of graft involvement. Positive predictive value of the functional imaging scans ranges between 80% to 90% in the detection of graft infection. False-positive results are not uncommon during the early postoperative period.

Endoscopy is very useful in cases of suspected secondary aortoenteric erosion or fistula and is an emergency procedure in patients with massive gastrointestinal bleeding where it can be performed in the operating theatre, with the patient prepared for operation. It is important is to visualize the third and fourth part of duodenum and rule out other sources of gastrointestinal bleeding. Though, an aortoduodenal fistula cannot be excluded by negative findings.

7. Operative findings

Operative exploration is sometimes mandatory for the final diagnosis, especially in unstable patients or in cases with a history of aortic grafting and gastrointestinal bleeding, where a GEF is suspected. Unfortunately only 50% of GEFs can be diagnosed by CT or MRI modalities. Operative exploration, graft excision and broth culture of the graft can lead to isolation of the responsible microorganisms and selection of proper antibiotic treatment.

8. Prevention

Prevention of graft contamination perioperatively is of great importance, given the high mortality and morbidity that follows a vascular infection. Antimicrobial prophylaxis should be administered within 60 min before incision and discontinued within 24 h after surgery. According to the published consensus of the Surgical Infection Prevention Guideline Writers Workgroup (SIPGWW), the recommended prophylactic antibiotics for cardiothoracic and vascular surgery include cefazolin and cefuroxime. [23] For intra-abdominal surgery coverage for anaerobes may be added (metronidazole). [24]

Culture-specific antibiotics should be administered to patients who have coexisting infections.

There are some principles that should be followed perioperatively, in order to prevent an infection:

- Patients should scrub the night before the operation
- Hair of the operative site should be removed by clippers and not by razors so as to prevent skin trauma
- Preoperative hospital stay should be minimized, if possible
- Remote infections must be controlled before elective grafting interventions
- Concomitant gastrointestinal procedures should be avoided, if a graft is planned to be used (cholecystectomy for asymptomatic cholelithiasis is possibly excepted)
- The use of iodine-impregnated plastic drapes is recommended, so as to prevent graft contamination
- Meticulous sterile technique is vital
- Careful hemostasis and closure of surgical incisions in multiple layers are recommended
- Irrigation of groin wounds with topical antibiotics before closure may decrease infection rates. [25]

9. Therapeutic management of vascular infection

9.1. General principles

Presentation of vascular infections varies and there is, usually, no standard treatment. Treatment should be individualized according to infection site, clinical presentation and the isolated microorganisms. For the extracavitary graft infections there are some recommendations, based on infection grade, simplifying the complexity of treatment. (Table 2) The main goal is eradication of the infection while preserving blood flow to the target organs or limbs.

Preparation of the patient is important, though takes time. In unstable patients due to septic or hypovolemic shock, no delay is justified. Blood or fluid resuscitation, antibiotic coverage and urgent surgical treatment are the only option. For the rest of the cases, where time is available, patient's cardiac, pulmonary and renal function should be optimized. Diabetic patients must have their glucose levels controlled. Malnourished patients can improve by enteral or parenteral nutrition. When an abdominal operation is planned, colon should be mechanically, cleansed. A Duplex scan of the lower limb veins is recommended, especially in cases of in situ replacement with autologous graft. Preoperative antibiotic coverage of the patient is crucial.

Available options include graft excision with or without revascularization and graft preservation with local treatment. Graft excision can be followed by extra anatomic revascularization or in situ replacement of the graft.

9.2. Preservation of the graft

Preservation of the infected graft is indicated in few, selected cases, usually when infection involves autologous vein grafts or patches. [26-28] Patients must have no signs of sepsis and the graft should be patent with segmental contamination. Anastomoses must be spared.

Outcome is better with vein or PTFE than polyester grafts, with early than late infections (<4 months) and with extracavitary grafts. Infections caused by single Gram positive and not multiple Gram negative organisms (e.g. Pseudomonas) may be considered for graft preservation and local treatment.

Local treatment includes staged surgical debridement of infected tissues in healthy plane, mechanical irrigation of the wound (using povidone iodine solution and peroxide), on a regular basis, rotational muscle flap coverage, temporary use of antibiotic impregnated beads and VAC devices (vacuum assisted closure devices for wounds). Intravenous culture-based antibiotics are essential. Persistent infection or sepsis is an indication of treatment failure which happens in 30% of the patients. [27] In such cases, graft excision with or without revascularization should follow.

9.3. Graft excision

Graft excision without revascularization is rarely an option, mostly in patients where the indication for the initial procedure was claudication, or in cases where the infection has led to graft thrombosis but with no signs of critical ischemia. In patent infected grafts, the decision regarding the need for immediate revascularization is based on temporary graft occlusion. The presence of Doppler pedal pulsatile signal and systolic ankle pressure greater than 40 mmHg is a sign of sufficient preexisting collaterals. In cases of infected bypass grafts with end to side anastomosis, the graft can be removed and an autologous patch can be placed at the site of proximal anastomosis.

In the majority of the cases, graft excision should be accompanied by revascularization of the target organs or limbs, usually by means of extra-anatomic PTFE bypass, through uninfected tissues.

This technique is suitable, mainly for aortoiliac or aortobifemoral infected grafts, for patients with GEE/GEF or for more diffuse infections with signs of systemic sepsis. Graft excision can be accomplished through celiotomy or left-side retroperitoneal incision, so as to avoid contaminated areas. Preoperative stenting of the ureters is recommended in cases of extensive infection, for protection during dissection and easier identification. Supraceliac aortic clamping and control of iliac arteries (at healthy segments, distally to the infected part of the graft) may be necessary, though sometimes difficult due to perigraft inflammation. Some centers advocate the use of intraluminal occlusion balloons. Meticulous dissection of the adherent viscera's or duodenum, especially in patients with GEE/GEF is important. Necrotic bowel segments must be excised and bowel continuity should be restored by end to end anastomosis. Complete removal and culture of the aortoiliofemoral graft must follow. Extensive debridement and irrigation (by use of cytotoxic agents) of perigraft contaminated or necrotic tissues are essential. Closure of the aortic stump is performed by double layers of interrupted monofilament sutures. Prosthetic pledgets should be avoided. Coverage of the aortic stump with omentum pedicles is believed to prevent stump blowout and its catastrophic consequences. The same technique can be applied for the ligation of iliac arteries, but flow must be maintained at least to one hypogastric artery, in order to avoid pelvic or colon ischemia. Placement of closed suction drains can be placed in the retroperitoneal space. Reported mortality rates range between 11-22%, while limb loss 10-11%. [20,29] Stump blowout, which is a major complication, can happen up to 22% of the cases. [7]

Several authors suggest that staged management of infected aortic grafts, show lower morbidity and mortality rates. [29,30] Hemodynamically unstable patients, are an exception, and the vascular surgeon should focus on the site of hemorrhage (septic hemorrhage from anastomosis, GEE/GEF). In the rest of the cases, it is recommended, to perform the extra-anatomic bypass first, and graft excision can follow 1 to 2 days later.

Aortobifemoral graft infections, especially in the groins, constitute a challenge for the surgeon. Unilateral ex situ bypass to the profunda femoris or superficial femoral artery through uninfected planes is an option, while bypass to the popliteal artery results in low rates of patency (58% in 6 months). [31] In bilateral groin infections, graft excision followed by unilateral axillofemoral bypass and autogenous vein cross-femoral bypass is another solution.

In-situ graft replacement is an alternative solution, in selected cases. There should be no systemic signs of sepsis, any anastomotic bleeding or perigraft incorporation. Perigraft fluid cultures must be sterile unless bacteria of low virulence, such as S. Epidermis, are isolated. In fact, in patients with infection that involves the thoracic aorta or the visceral segment of abdominal aorta, in situ replacement may be the only option available. The most common grafts used in this technique are autologous grafts (e.g. superficial or deep veins of the limbs), antibiotic bonded prosthetic grafts or cryopreserved arterial allografts. (Figure 1.)

Great saphenous vein (GSV) or superficial veins from the upper limb can be used in cases where infection affects infrainguinal, upper extremity, visceral or cerebrovascular procedures. A preoperative Duplex vein mapping is essential for estimation of vein's condition and diameter.

However, use of GSV in ilio-femoral or aorto-iliac reconstructions, results in low patency rates, due to diameter mismatch. [32] In these cases, superficial femoral vein harvesting has a strong indication. [33,34] Preoperative vein mapping is important. In cases of aortic reconstruction, with larger aortic diameter, "pantaloon technique" can be applied. (Figure 1.) Compared to graft excision and extra anatomic bypass, in situ graft replacement presents better patency and recurrent infection rates. [35] Superficial femoral vein can be used also, in aortofemoral graft infections localized in the groin caused by S. epidermidis. However its use in secondary GEE/GEF is not recommended. Deep veins are used non reversed, after valve excision.

Antibiotic bonded prosthetic grafts (PTFE or Dacron), can be used in segmental graft infections, where the isolated microorganism is of low virulence (e.g. S. Epidermidis) and the anastomoses are spared. [20] For example in segmental aortofemoral graft infections, with groin complications, especially in elderly patients, antibiotic bonded prosthetic grafts should be considered for replacement of one limb of the pre-existing graft.

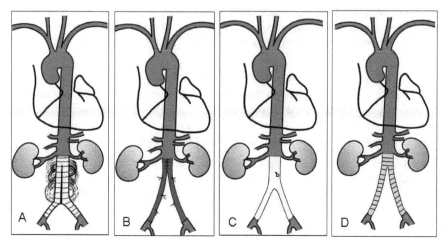

Figure 1. In situ aortic reconstruction after graft infection (A= infected bifurcated graft, B= autologous replacement ("Pantaloon" technique),   C= heterologous replacement (bovine aorta),D= Repair with silver-bonded synthetic graft)

An alternative option, especially in more diffuse infections, is the use of cryopreserved arterial allografts. While the survival and recurrent infection rates are comparable to other grafts, increased dilation (17%) and stenosis (20%) rates were noticed. [36]

Overall, outcomes following deep venous replacement are better than with the use of arterial allografts or implantation of a "new" prosthetic graft. When applied to low-grade aortic graft infections without GEE or GEF, this procedure is safe (4% in-hospital mortality), with a low (3%) incidence of long-term limb loss. In cases with GEE/GEF, mortality can reach 20%, similar to graft excision and ex-situ bypass.

10. Adjunctive treatments

10.1. Antibiotic-loaded beads

In vascular infections, where graft preservation and serial debridement of the wound is the selected treatment, implantation of antibiotic –loaded beads is an alternative adjunctive therapy. They are mainly used in extracavitary graft infections. Beads are usually loaded with vancomycin, daptomycin, tobramycin, or gentamicin based on initial culture results. Initial results are encouraging, with wound healing in 90% of the cases. [37]

10.2. Muscle flap coverage

Infected grafts that are treated locally must be surrounded by healthy, non contaminated tissues. Coverage of the graft with a well vascularised, not infected muscle flap, contributes to wound healing. Sartorius muscle flap coverage is the most common technique used in graft infections located in the groins. [38] This technique is mainly indicated, as an adjunct of graft preservation or in situ replacement therapies, especially in cases of recurrent infections or extensive tissue deficit after debridement. The muscle is divided from its proximal attachment to the iliac crest and sutured medially, so as to cover the infected graft. In a published series, recurrent infection rate after use of Sartorius flap was only 7%. [39]

Another similar technique is the rotational use of flaps of muscles that are mobilized from a separate healthy site. Their blood supply doesn't come from the infected area. The gracilis rectus abdominis, tensor fasciae latae or rectus femoris can be used, depending on site of infection. [40] Some authors consider this technique as a better option than the use of Sartorius muscle. [38]

10.3. Antibiotics

When the diagnosis of vascular infection is made, parenteral broad spectrum antibiotics should be given, until isolation of the infecting micro-organism is accomplished, through cultures. Additionally, if cultures reveal no pathogen or there are no available specimens for culture, empiric antimicrobial treatment should target skin-colonizing organisms and nosocomial pathogens as well.

Vancomycin is an indispensable agent in the initial empiric antimicrobial regimen, because of its excellent anti-Gram-positive spectrum. Teicoplanin has a similar antimicrobial spectrum to vancomycin but has not been tested in large prospective series for the treatment of vascular infections. [41-44]

Alternative antimicrobial agents are linezolid and quinupristin/dalfopristin, which provide coverage for methicillin-resistant staphylococci (MRSA and MRSE) and vancomycin-resistant enterococci (VRE). Their use should be reserved for infections due to pathogens resistant to vancomycin, or in patients who are allergic to vancomycin. [45,46]

Once cultures reveal the infecting pathogen , parenteral antibiotic treatment should be initiated, without any delay.

The duration of therapy is individualized but most authors recommend 4–6 weeks of treatment after the removal of the infected graft.

11. Management of specific graft site infection

11.1. Carotid infection

Depending on grading, carotid artery infections are reported up to 2% of cases. [47] Szylagyi III infections are found in a rate of less than 1%. [48,49] The majority of infections are postoperative wound contaminations, which seldom extent to the suture line. Wound dehiscence with septic haemorrhage is extremely rarely observed. There are reports that the use of prosthetic materials increases the infection rate. However, the management of such infections that may lead to catastrophic life-threatening septic complications is especially challenging. The standard treatment includes wound debridement and prosthetic graft replacement with autologous material (e.g. saphenous vein). Recently the use of sternocleidomastoid muscle flap plasty for coverage of the infected area was described. More recently, carotid stent infections were reported in up to 0,4 % of cases. [48] This complication may present primary or secondary to neck irradiation and trauma. [48,50,51] The treatment principles are similar to post-CEA infections. The use of vacuum assisted closure device emerges as a new trend with promising results. [52]

11.2. Infection of vascular access

Vascular access Infection is a major complication for haemodialysis patients. Clinical symptoms vary from simple local inflammation to systemic sepsis. In some cases, septic haemorrhage may develop, which is a life-threatening condition. (Figure 2.) Reported risk factors for this adverse event include immunodeficiency, low serum albumin level, female gender, adult polycystic kidney disease, diabetes mellitus, inadequate dialysis and the use of catheters or synthetic graft. [53] It is estimated that 30 to 50% of bacteraemia in haemodialysis patients is caused by vascular access infection. [53] There are reports that infection rates range from 0.5 to 3.5% for autogenous AVF, 5-8% for prosthetic graft accesses and 2-5.5 episodes of bacteremia per 1000 patient days for central venous catheters. [54,55]

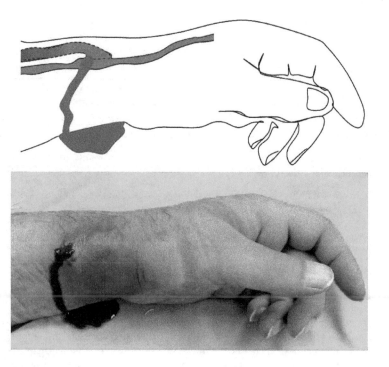

Figure 2. Infection of brachio-cephalic fistula (Cimino) at the wrist with septic bleeding

Early postoperative graft infections usually affect the whole graft. The treatment of choice is excision of the entire graft. Late localised infection at the needles sites can be managed by segmental graft removal and bypass through uninfected planes. Sometimes, though, total excision is necessary.

The use of V.A.C. as an adjunctive treatment may be beneficial. Autogenous AV access infections often can be effectively treated with systemic antibiotics. In case of infected pseudoaneurysms or abscesses access ligation of the access or segmental bypass are mandatory.

Catheter infection presentation varies. Exit-site infections are treated with local antibiotics. In case of failure, parenteral antibiotics should be administered. Tunnel tract infections require intravenous antibiotics, and catheter exchange through a new tunnel and exit site. These patients require at least 3 weeks of culture-based antibiotic therapy and monitoring for recurrent infection. [56] Patients with systemic sepsis should have their catheter removed and a temporary catheter inserted. A new cuffed catheter may be placed if the patient remains afebrile for at least 48-72 hours.

11.3. Infection of thoracic aorta

The incidence of infections affecting thoracic or thoracoabdominal aortic grafts, ranges from 0.5% to 1.9%. Complications can be fatal, and mortality is high. Open surgical repair for primary or secondary thoracic aorta infections are associated with significant mortality and morbidity. Graft excision and extra-anatomic bypass are usually not applicable to infections involving ascending, transverse arch or descending aorta grafts. For most of these cases, in-situ replacement with the use of prosthetic grafts is the treatment of choice. The use of silver-bonded or antimicrobial-bonded synthetic grafts is possibly preferable. Surgical debridement and antibacterial irrigation of infected tissues are important. It is reported that coverage of the graft with pericardial fat, rotated muscles (e.g. pectoralis major, latissimus dorsi, rectus abdominis) or with a pedicle of greater omentum can prevent recurrent infections. [57] Antibiotic coverage is necessary. Mortality is reported to be 10-20% while reinfection rates 20%. [57,58] The only extra-anatomic repair, that may be recommended, is prosthetic grafting from the ascending to abdominal aorta, tunnelling through the diaphragm, with subsequent infected graft excision through a left thoracotomy. Limited surgical strategy involving extensive mediastinal debridement is reported in cases where infection is associated with sternal wound infection by low virulent pathogens. [59] Endovascular stent graft repair has been reported as an attractive and effective treatment option, but the persistence of infection is always a concern. Though in cases of severe local inflammation, with or without haemorrhage, this technique can serve as bridging therapy. [60]

Stent or stent-graft infections in the thoracic aorta are extremely rare. They are usually met in the literature as complications of systemic specific infections such as TBC or brucellosis. The general principles of treatment are similar to the thoracic graft infection. Some papers report secondary stent-graft infections after TEVAR due to aorto-oesophageal or aorto-bronchial fistulas.

11.4. Vascular infections in the groin

Infections after vascular reconstructions are most common in the groins. The main predisposing factors are surgical division of lymphatic channels, infected lymph glands, the superficial location of vascular grafts and the proximity of the surgical site to the perineum. A number of serious complications can arise such as fistula, septic hemorrhage, septic embolism and limb threatening ischemia. [61,62] Imaging of the infected area is essential for the diagnosis. (Figure 3.)

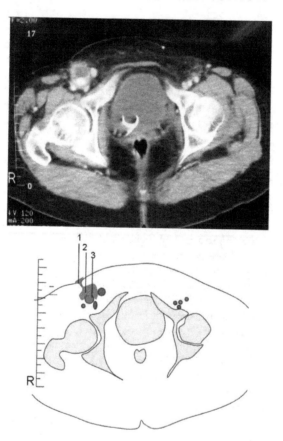

Figure 3. CT findings in a patient with Szilagyi III infection in the groin. (1=fistula, 2=perigraft inflammation/secretion, 3=graft)

There is a lot of controversy about the treatment of choice in groin infections, following vascular graft placement. It depends on the degree of graft involvement. If there is no graft infection (Szilagyi grade I or II), then wound debridement or drainage with culture-directed antibiotic administration is considered to be adequate. If, graft contamination is present

(Szilagyi grade III), then further treatment is controversial. In the majority of the cases, treatment includes excision of the graft, surgical debridement of the infected tissues followed by restoration of blood flow by in situ or extra-anatomic reconstruction.[63,64] Obturator or lateral femoral bypass are the most frequent extra-anatomic procedures for limb revascularization in vascular groin infections. [65-67] An 80% cumulative patency rate at 6 years has been reported. [68] However, many concerns have been associated to extra-anatomic bypass including lengthy procedure time, difficulty of extra-anatomic routing, high amputation rates. [69]. When in-situ reconstruction is selected, cryopreserved aortic homograft, autologous deep femoral vein, or rifampin-bonded prostheses can serve as grafts. Disadvantages associated with in situ reconstructions, include lengthier operative time in case of vein harvesting and contraindication in patients with previous deep vein thrombosis, high complication rates of cryopreserved allografts and lack of availability in emergent cases. In situ reconstructions are associated with higher stress than extra-anatomic bypasses, which is important in high risk patients.

Graft preservation is considered an option when the graft is patent, the entire length of the graft is not involved by the infection, the anastomosis is intact, there are no systemic signs of sepsis and the contaminating organism is not a virulent strain of bacteria, especially MRSA and Pseudomonas aeruginosa . [70,71]

The use of local muscle flaps to promote wound healing and vascular graft salvage has been well documented. [72-74]

VAC therapy has been reported as an adjunctive or definitive treatment for groin infections involving exposed grafts especially in high-risk surgical patients who are not candidates for graft replacement. VAC therapy along with aggressive debridement, antibiotic therapy and muscle flap coverage may be an effective alternative to current management strategies. Some authors recommend the use of V.A.C. even after graft replacement, in treatment of Szilagyi III infections. (Figure 4.)

The majority of current clinical evidence supporting the use of negative pressure therapy (VAC) on infected groin wounds following vascular reconstructions has been based on clinical experience and small cohort studies. However graft/patch salvage rates up to 97.2%, have been reported. [75].

11.5. Infection of femoral, popliteal, tibial grafts

Infection of infrainguinal grafts is quite rare but it can present with anastomotic disruption and septic hemorrhage or emboli. The preferred method of treatment is usually graft excision and revascularization with bypass grafting via adjacent or remote tunneling. In-situ revascularization is feasible in 80% of the cases. The use of autogenous vein grafts is preferred when they are available. Some authors advocate staged treatment. In this case, closure of the arteriotomies with monofilament suture and the administration of systemic and topical antibiotics follow the removal of the graft. Patients who had prosthetic grafts inserted for claudication or patients who do not develop limb-threatening ischemia after graft excision may not need revascularization.

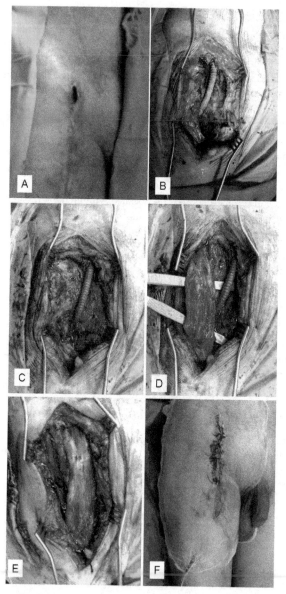

Figure 4. Application of vacuum-assisted closure technique (VAC technique) in a patient with graft infection in groin (A=Szilagyi III infection with cutaneous fistula, B=marking of infected area with use of methylene blue, C=Wound debridement and replacement of infected graft with a silver-bonded synthetic graft, D=preparation of sartorius muscle, E= coverage of the graft with the muscle flap, D=Application of VAC system

Graft preservation is reported as an alternative option, especially in high risk patients, unless there is sepsis or anastomotic bleeding. In such cases local treatment with surgical debridement, antibiotic administration and muscle flap coverage is applied. [19,30]

Treatment of peripheral grafts infection shows low mortality rates (0-9%) but increased amputation rates (33-67%) compared to treatment of aortic grafts infection. [11,76]

11.6. Endovascular stent-graft and stent infections

Infections involving endoluminal devices (stents or stent-grafts) are rare, although they present with increased frequency. The reported incidence after AAA repair is 0.2% to 1.2%. Infection of peripheral bare stents are extremely rare (<0.1%). They present clinically with sepsis, septic emboli, mycotic aneurysm or GEE/GEF. Periprocedural bacteremia from remote sites of infection or during secondary endovascular interventions is considered to be the cause of stent-graft contamination. [77] Perigraft inflammation or fluid is the main CT findings with diagnostic sensitivity of 85%. Treatment consists of antibiotics and graft excision followed by extra-anatomic bypass or in situ autogenous replacement. Mortality is high and ranges between 20-30%. [78,79] Endovascular treatment should be considered only as a bridging therapy. [80,81]

Author details

Kiriakos Ktenidis* and Argyrios Giannopoulos

1st Department of Surgery, Aristotle University of Thessaloniki, Greece

12. References

[1] Szilagyi DE, et al. Infection in arterial reconstruction with synthetic grafts. Ann Surg. 1972;176(3):321-33.

[2] Karl T, Storck M. Indikationen der V.A.C. ®- Therapie bei der Behandlung von postoperativen Wundheilungsstörungen nach alloplastischer Bypassimplantation. Eine modifizierte Klassifikation. Vasomed 2010;22: 160-63.

[3] Samson RH, et al. A modified classification and approach to the management of infections involving peripheral arterial prosthetic grafts. J Vasc Surg. 1988;8(2):147-53.

[4] Bandyk DF. Vascular graft infections: Epidemiology, microbiology, pathogenesis, and prevention. In: Bernhard VM, Towne JB (eds): Complications in Vascular Surgery. St. Louis: Quality Medical; 1991. p 223–234.

[5] Bunt TJ. Synthetic vascular graft infections. Surgery 1988.;93:733.

[6] Fry WJ, Lindenauer SM. Infection complicating the use of plastic arterial implants. Arch Surg 1966; 94:600.

[7] O'Hara PJ, Hertzer NR, Beven EG, et al. Surgical management of infected abdominal aortic grafts: Review of a 25-year experience. J Vasc Surg 1986.;3:725.

* Corresponding Author

[8] Hallett JW, Marshall DM, Petterson TM, et al. Graft-related complications after abdominal aortic aneurysm repair: Population-based experience. J Vasc Surg 1977;25:277.

[9] Bandyk DF. Infection of prosthetic vascular grafts. In:Rutherford RB (ed): Vascular Surgery, 5th ed. St. Louis: CV Mosby; 1995. p 566.

[10] Campbell WB, Tambeeur LJ, Geens VR. Local complications after arterial bypass grafting. Ann R Coll Surg Engl 1994;76:127.

[11] Liekweg WG Jr, Greenfield LJ. Vascular prosthetic infections: Collected experience and results of treatment. Surgery 1977; 81:335.

[12] Naylor AR, Payne D, London NJ, et al. Prosthetic patch infection after carotid endarterectomy. Eur J Vasc Surg 2002;23:11.

[13] Ohki T, Veith FJ, Shaw P, et al. Increasing incidence of midterm and long-term complications after endovascular graft repair of abdominal aortic aneurysms: A note of caution based on a 9-year experience. Ann Surg 2001;234:323.

[14] Deiparine MK, Ballard JL, Taylor FC, Chase DR. Endovascular stent infection. J Vasc Surg 1996;23:529.

[15] Darling RC III, Resnikoff M, Kreienberg PB, et al. Alternative approach for management of infected aortic grafts. J Vasc Surg 1997;25:106.

[16] Bandyk DF, Berni GA, Thiele BL, et al. Aortofemoral graft infection due to Staphylococcus epidermidis. Arch Surg 1984;119:102.

[17] Olofsson PA, Auffermann W, Higgins CB, et al. Diagnosis of prosthetic aortic graft infection by magnetic resonance imaging. J Vasc Surg 1988; 8:99.

[18] Calligaro KD, Veith FJ, Schwartz ML, et al. Differences in early versus late extracavitary arterial graft infections. J Vasc Surg 1995;22:680.

[19] Calligaro KD, Veith FJ, Yuan JG, et al. Intra-abdominal aortic graft infection: Complete or partial graft preservation in patients at very high risk. J Vasc Surg 2003;38:1199.

[20] Bandyk DF, Novotney ML, Back MR. Expanded application of in situ replacement for prosthetic graft infection. J Vasc Surg 2001;34:411.

[21] Schmitt DD, Seabrook GR, Bandyk DF, et al. Graft excision and extra-anatomic revascularization: The treatment of choice for the septic aortic prosthesis. J Cardiovasc Surg 1990;31:327.

[22] Walker WE, Cooley DA, Duncan JM, et al. The management of aortoduodenal fistula by in situ replacement of the infected abdominal aortic graft. Ann Surg 1987;205:727.

[23] Anonymous. Antimicrobial prophylaxis in surgery. Med Lett Drugs Ther 2001; 43:92–97

[24] Talbot TR, Kaiser AB Postoperative infections and antimicrobial prophylaxis. In:Mandell GL, Bennett JE, Dolin R (eds) Principles and practice of infectious diseases, 6th edn. Churchill Livingstone, New York,;2005. 33–3547.

[25] Bergamini TM, Bandyk DF, Govostis D, et al. Identification of Staphylococcus epidermidis vascular graft infections: A comparison of culture techniques. J Vasc Surg 1989;9:665.

[26] Calligaro KD, Westcott CJ, Buckley RM, et al. Infrainguinal anastomotic arterial graft infections treated by selective graft preservation. Ann Surg 1993.;216:74.

[27] Calligaro KD, Veith FJ, Schwartz ML, et al. Selective preservation of infected prosthetic grafts: Analysis of a 20-year experience with 120 extra-cavitary infected grafts. Ann Surg 1994;220:461.

[28] Calligaro KD, Veith FJ, Schwartz ML, et al. Are gram-negative bacteria a contraindication to selective preservation of infected prosthetic arterial grafts? J Vasc Surg 1992; 16:337.

[29] Seeger JM, Pretus HA, Welborn MB, et al. Long-term outcome after treatment of aortic graft infection with staged extra-anatomic bypass and aortic graft removal. J Vasc Surg 2000;32:451.

[30] Reilly LM, Stoney RJ, Goldstone J, et al. Improved management of aortic graft infection: The influence of operation sequence and staging. J Vasc Surg 1987; 5:421.

[31] Seeger JM, Back MR, Albright JL, et al. Influence of patient characteristics and treatment options on outcome of patients with prosthetic aortic graft infection. Ann Vasc Surg 1999; 13:413.

[32] Seeger JM, Wheeler JR, Gregory RT, et al. Autogenous graft replacement of infected prosthetic grafts in the femoral position. Surgery 1983; 93:39.

[33] Clagett GP, Bowers BL, Lopez-Viego MA, et al. Creation of a neo-aortoiliac system from lower extremity deep and superficial veins. Ann Surg 1993; 218:239.

[34] Nevelsteen A, Lacroix H, Suy R. Autogenous reconstruction of the lower extremity deep veins: an alternative treatment of prosthetic infection after reconstructive surgery of aortoiliac disease. J Vasc Surg 1995; 22:129.

[35] Clagett GP, Valentine RJ, Hagino RT. Autogenous aortoiliac/femoral reconstruction from superficial femoral-popliteal veins: feasibility and durability. J Vasc Surg 1997; 25:25.

[36] Kieffer E, Gomes D, Chiche L, et al. Allograft replacement for infrarenal aortic graft infection: early and late results in 179 patients. J Vasc Surg 2004; 39:1009.

[37] Stone PA, Armstrong PA, Bandyk DF, et al. Use of antibiotic-loaded polymethylmethacrylate beads for the treatment of extra-cavitary prosthetic graft infection. J Vasc Surg 2006; 44:757.

[38] Perler BA, Vanderkolk CA, Manson PM, et al. Rotational muscle flaps to treat localized prosthetic graft infection: long-term follow-up. J Vasc Surg 1993; 18:358.

[39] Armstrong PA, Back MR, Bandyk DF, et al. Selective application of sartorius muscle flaps and aggressive staged surgical debridement can influence long-term outcomes of complex prosthetic graft infections. J Vasc Surg 2007; 46:71.

[40] Mathes SSJ, McGrow JB, Vasconez LO. Muscle transposition flaps for coverage of lower extremity deficits. Anatomic considerations. Surg Clin North Am 1954;54:1337.

[41] Antrum RM, Galvin K, Gorst K et al. Teicoplanin vs cephradine and metronidazole in the prophylaxis of sepsisfollowing vascular surgery: an interim analysis of an ongoingtrial. Eur J Surg Suppl 1992;567:43–46.

[42] Giacometti A, Cirioni O, Ghiselli R et al. Vascular graft infection by Staphylococcus epidermidis: efficacy of various perioperative prophylaxis protocols in an animal model. Infez Med 2001; 9:13–18.

[43] Gilbert DN, Wood CA, Kimbrough RC. Failure of treatment with teicoplanin at 6 milligrams/kilogram/day in patients with Staphylococcus aureus intravascular infection. The Infectious Diseases Consortium of Oregon; 1991.

[44] Antimicrob Agents C Kester RC, AntrumR,Thornton CA et al. A comparison of teicoplanin versus cephradine plus metronidazole in the prophylaxis of post-operative infection in vascular surgery. J Hosp Infect 1999;41:233–243.

[45] Antonios VS, Baddour LM. Intra-arterial device infections. Curr Infect Dis Rep 2004;6:263–269.

[46] Baddour LM, Bettman MA, Bolger AF et al. Nonvalvular cardiovascular device-related infections. Circulation 2003; 108:2015–2031.

[47] Ferguson GG, Eliasziw M, Barr HW, Clagett GP, Barnes RW, Wallace MC, et al. The North American Symptomatic Carotid Endarterectomy Trial : surgical results in 1415 patients. Stroke 1999;30(9) 1751-1758.

[48] Mas JL for for the EVA-3S Investigators. Endarterectomy versus Angioplasty in Patients with Symptomatic Severe Carotid Stenosis (EVA-3S) N Engl J Med 2006;355:1660-71.

[49] Naylor A.R. et al. Prosthetic Patch Infection After Carotid Endarterectomy Eur J Vasc Endovasc Surg 2002;23(1) 11–16.

[50] Kaviani A, Ouriel M, Kashyap VS. Infected carotid pseudoaneurysm and carotid-cutaneous fistula as a late complication of carotid artery stenting. J Vasc Surg 2006;43:379–382.

[51] Desai JA, Husain SF, Islam O, Jin AY. Carotid artery stent infection with Streptococcus agalactiae. Neurology. 2010;74(4):344.

[52] Kragsterman B, Björck M, Wanhainen A. EndoVAC, a novel hybrid technique to treat infected vascular reconstructions with an endograft and vacuum-assisted wound closure. J Endovasc Ther 2011;18(5):666-73.

[53] Tokars JI, Light P, Anderson J, et al. A prospective study of vascular access infections at seven outpatient haemodialysis centers. Am J Kidney Dis 2001;37 :1232-1240.

[54] Beathard GA. Management of bacteremia associated with tunneled-cuffed hemodialysis catheters. J Am Soc Nephrol 1999;10:1045– 1049.

[55] Saad TF: Bacteremia associated with tunneled, cuffed hemodialysis catheters. Am J Kidney Dis 1999; 34:1114–1124.

[56] Robinson D., Suhocki P., Schwab SJ. Treatmentof infected tunnelled venous accesshemodialysis catheters with guidewire exchange. Kidney Int 1998;53:1792-4.

[57] Coselli JS, Crawford ES, Williams TW, et al. Treatment of postoperative infection of ascending aorta and transverse aortic arch, including use of viable omentum and muscle flaps. Ann Thorac Surg 1990;50:868.

[58] Kieffer E, Sabatier J, Plissonnier D, et al. Prosthetic graft infection after descending thoracic/thoracoabdominal aortic aneurysmectomy: management with in situ arterial grafts. J Vasc Surg 2001; 33:671.

[59] Akowuah E, Narayan P Jr, Angelini G, Bryan AJ. Management of prosthetic graft infection after surgery of the thoracic aorta: removal of the prosthetic graft is not necessary. J Thorac Cardiovasc Surg. 2007;134:1051-2.

[60] Ting AC, Cheng SW, Ho P, Poon JT.Endovascular stent graft repair for infected thoracic aortic pseudoaneurysms--a durable option?J Vasc Surg 2006;44(4) 701-5.

[61] Atnip RG. Crossover ilioprofunda reconstruction: an expanded role for obturator foramen bypass. Surgery 1991;110:106-8.

[62] Patel KR, Semel L, Clauss RH. Routine revascularization with resection of infection femoral pseudoaneurysms from substance abuse. J Vasc Surg 1988;8:321-8.

[63] Bandyk DF. Infection in prosthetic vascular grafts. In: Rutherford RB, (ed.) Vascular surgery. 5th ed. Philadelphia: WB Saunders; 2000.p733-51.

[64] Reddy DJ, Ernst CB. Infected aneurysms. In: Rutherford RB, (ed.) Vascular surgery. 5th ed. Philadelphia: WB Saunders; 2000.p1383-97.

[65] Donahoe PK, Froio RA, Nabseth DC. Obturator bypass graft in radical excision of inguinal neoplasm. Ann Surg 1967;166:147-9.

[66] Favre JP, Gournier JP, Barral X. Trans-osseous ilio-femoral by-pass. A new extra-anatomical by-pass. J Cardiovasc Surg (Torino) 1993;34:455-9.

[67] Brzezinski W, Callaghan JC. Transiliac bypass for infected femoral end of an aortofemoral graft. Can J Surg 1989;32:121-3.

[68] van Det RJ, Brands LC. The obturator foramen bypass: an alternative procedure in iliofemoral artery revascularization. Surgery 1981;89:543-7.

[69] O'Connor S., Peter Andrew P., Michel Batt M., Becquemin J. P. A systematic review and meta-analysis of treatments for aortic graft infection. J Vasc Surg 2006;44:38-45.

[70] Dosluoglu H. H., Schimpf D. K., Schultz R. et al. Preservation of infected and exposed vascular grafts using vacuum assisted closure without muscle flap coverage. J Vasc Surg 2005;42:989-92.

[71] Calligaro K. D., Veith F. J., Sales C. M. et al. Comparison of muscle flaps and delayed secondary intention wound healing for infected lower extremity arterial grafts. Ann Vasc Surg 1994;8:31-7.

[72] Mixter R. C., Turnipseed W. D., Smith D. J. Jr. et al. Rotational muscle flaps:a new technique for covering infected vascular grafts. J Vasc Surg 1989;9:472-8.

[73] Mckenna P. J., Leadbetter M. G. Salvage of chronically exposed Gore-Tex vascular access grafts in the hemodialysis patient. Plast Reconstr Surg 1988;82:1046-51.

[74] Perler B. A., Vander Kolk C. A., Dufresne C. R. et al. Can infected prosthetic grafts be salvaged with rotational muscle flaps ? Surgery 1991;110:30-4.

[75] Ktenidis K., Tripathi R.:Case study Vacuum Assisted Closure® (V.A.C.®) Therapy for Vascular Graft Infection (Szilagyi Grade III) in the Groin - A Ten-Year Multi-Center Experience. J Vasc Surg 2010,51:12S-12S.

[76] Durham JR, Rubin JR, Malone JM. Management of infected infrainguinal bypass grafts. In: Bergan JJ, Yao JST (eds): Reoperative Arterial Surgery. Orlando, FL, Grune & Stratton; 1986,p359–373.

[77] Pruitt A, Dodson TF, Najibi S, et al. Distal septic emboli and fatal brachiocephalic artery mycotic pseudoaneurysm as a complication of stenting. J Vasc Surg 2002;36:625.

[78] Alankar S, Barth MH, Shin DD, et al. Aortoduodenal fistula and associated rupture of abdominal aortic aneurysm after endoluminal stent-graft repair. J Vasc Surg 2003;37:465.

[79] Jackson MR, Joiner DR, Clagett GP. Excision and autogenous revascularization of an infected aortic stent graft resulting from a urinary tract infection. J Vasc Surg 2002;36:622.

[80] Curti T, Freyrie A, Mirelli M, et al. Endovascular treatment of an ilioenteric fistula: a bridge to aortic homograft. Eur J Vasc Endovasc Surg 2000;20:204.

[81] Chuter TAM, Lukaszewicz GC, Reilly LM, et al. Endovascular repair of a presumed aortoenteric fistula: late failure due to recurrent infection. J Endovasc Ther 2000;7:240.

Peripheral Artery Disease and Varicose Vein

Chapter 4

Day Case Management of Varicose Veins

Jesus Barandiaran, Thomas Hall, Naif El-Barghouti and Eugene Perry

Additional information is available at the end of the chapter

1. Introduction

Lower limb varicose veins are a common disease that affects almost a quarter of the adult population. They are one of the commonest conditions requiring intervention. They affect women more frequently than men, and are reported in 20-60% of the general population. Approximately one million people in the United Kingdom are affected with VV. Nearly half a million seek advice from their primary care practitioner about VV in the lower limbs and their related symptoms every year. Of those, 75,000 patients receive some form of intervention. It is estimated that surgical treatment of varicose veins are responsible for 54000 hospital episodes per year in England. They constitute a large part of elective surgical waiting lists [1, 2 and 3].

The treatment of primary varicose veins is considered appropriate by the majority of vascular surgeons if the veins are symptomatic. Common symptoms include poor cosmesis, aching and itching. Less common problems are haemorrhage, thrombophlebitis, ankle pigmentation, lipodermosclerosis and ulceration. The extent of visible veins does not correlate with the severity of the symptoms experienced by patients [4].

Treatment options available for varicose veins traditionally included either conservative management with lifestyle advice and compression hosiery or surgery. Surgery involves saphenofemoral junction disconnection and stripping of the long saphenous vein and multiple stab avulsions for varicose veins stemming from saphenofemoral reflux; saphenopopliteal disconnection for saphenopopliteal reflux [2].

Results from traditional surgery are excellent and have stood the test of time. However, there has been an expansion of less invasive treatment modalities for VV, such as radiofrequency ablation, endovenous laser treatment, sclerotherapy (liquid and foam), transilluminated powered phlebectomy, and subfascial endoscopic perforator vein surgery. These minimally invasive therapies are attractive to both patients and healthcare professionals but there is paucity of good quality data from randomized control trials [5].

Moreover, the need for specialized equipment and additional training to become proficient at new techniques, prevent surgeons from practicing these procedures.

In the United Kingdom, until there is long-term follow-up with the less invasive procedures, the gold standard for VV surgery is still a standard saphenofemoral junction ligation and disconnection (SFJLD) with stripping of the long saphenous vein and multiple stab avulsions. As stripping of the long saphenous vein is painful, this surgery requires a general anaesthetic and an overnight in-patient stay for satisfactory recovery.

We propose a new approach to addressing problems with VV in the lower limb that obviates the need for a general anaesthesia. After SFJLD, the varicosities in the long saphenous system are rarely fed retrogradely unless there are incompetent perforators— thus, varicosities in the lower limb would be expected to diminish in size and length. If the long saphenous vein is left in situ without stripping and stab avulsions are not done at the time of groin exploration for SFJLD, VV surgery can be done safely under local anaesthetic. Currently, we perform multiple stab avulsions (under local anaesthetic) as a second-stage procedure at 6 months post-SFJLD.

The purpose of this study was twofold. The first aim was to study the longitudinal functional and cosmetic outcome in a consecutive series of patients who had SFJLD under local anaesthetic. Our second aim was to identify the optimum time gap from SFJLD to multiple stab avulsions for residual VV.

2. Methods

A prospective observational study was designed by the Scarborough General Hospital Vascular team. It was carried out between June 2006 and June 2008.

The patients were recruited in two different out patient clinics, including Scarborough General Hospital Outpatient department and Malton County Hospital Outpatient Department. Both clinics were supervised by a single Consultant Vascular Surgeon.

A very specific inclusion criteria was devised to select the patients to be included in this study:

1. Patients met the National Institute of Clinical Excelence guidelines for treatment of Varicose Veins.
2. Patients with clinical evidence of Primary varicose veins of the Long Saphenous Vein distribution.
3. All patients had clinical and ultrasonographic evidence of incompetence at the Saphenofemoral junction. This was demonstrated using, either a Hand Held Doppler Machine or a Venous Duplex Ultrasound Scan.
4. All patients were suitable for Local Anaesthetic Surgery in a day case setting
   - Patients had a BMI less than 35
   - Patients had transport arranged to go back home as they were not allowed to drive themselves

- Patients had a responsible carer to look after them postoperatively
- Patients were ASA (American Society of Anaesthesiologist Classification) I, II or III
- Patient/Carer must have access to a private telephone
- Patients residence must be within one and a half hour of a Hospital with Accident and Emergency and Vascular facilities

Exclusion criteria included

1. Pregnancy
2. Age below 18 years
3. Allergy to Local Anaesthetic Agents
4. Patients with Varicose veins of the Short Saphenous System distribution
5. Recurrent Varicose Veins
6. Patients with complex varicosities
7. Previous history of Deep Vein Thromboembolis
8. Areas of active ulceration (CEAP Classification C6)

2.1. Veins and questionnaire assessment

Suitable patients were seen preoperatively in the Outpatient Clinic. All the visible varicose veins were marked with a permanent ink pen. After that, the length of varicosities was measured using a cartographer's wheel (Figure 1)

The outer ring of the cartographer's ring measures the length of varicosities in centimetres and gives us an accurate measurement of the extension of the Varicose Veins. This measurement was done by a single assessor.

A higher measurement on the wheel cartograph meant a greater volume of varicose veins.

Every patient taking part in the trial was asked to fill up four standardized health questionnaires:

1. CEAP score

Mark	DEFINITION
C	Clinical signs (grade 0-6) supplemented by (s) for symptomatic and (a) for asymptomatic presentation
E	Ethiological Classification (Congenital, Primary, Secondary)
A	Anatomical Distribution (Superficial, Deep, Perforator)
P	Pathophysiology Dysfunction (Reflux, Obstruction)

Table 1. Classification of chronic lower extremity venous disease. CEAP score

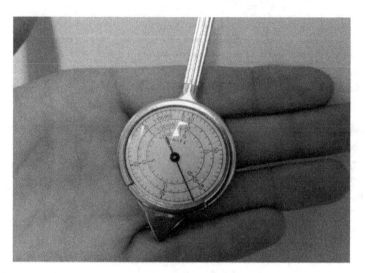

Figure 1.

Class	Cinical signs
0	No visible or palpable signs of venous disease
1	Telangiectases, reticular veins, malleolar flare
2	Varicose Veins
3	Oedema without skin changes
4	Skin changes ascribed to venous disease (pigmentation,venous eczema, lipodermatosclerosis)
5	Skin changes in conjunction with healed ulceration
6	Skin changes in conjunction with active ulceration

Table 2. CEAP Clinical classification of chronic lower extremity venous disease

2. Venous clinical severity score

Attribute	Absent = 0	Mild = 1	Moderate = 2	Severe = 3
Pain	None	Occasional	Daily	Limit activities
Varicose veins	None	Few, scattered	Multiple (LSV)	Extensive (LSV, SSV)
Venous Oedema	None	Evening, Ankle	Afternoon, leg	Morning, leg
Pigmentation	None	Limited area	Wide (lower 1/3)	Wider (Above 1/3)
Inflamation	None	Cellulitis	Cellulitis	Cellulitis
Induration	None	Focal (<5 cm)	<lower 1/3	Entire lower 1/3
Number of AC	None	1	2	3
Duration of AC	None	<3 months	3 months- 1 year	>1 year
Size of AC	None	<2 cm diameter	2-6 cm diameter	>6 cm diameter
Comp therapy	Not used	Intermittent use	Most days	Continually

3. Aberdeen varicose vein severity score

1. Please draw in your varicose veins in the diagram below: Vein grid
2. In the last two weeks, for how many days did your varicose veins cause you pain or ache?
3. during the last two weeks, on how many days did you take painkilling tablets for your varicose veins?
4. In the last two weeks, how much ankle swelling have you had?
5. In the last two weeks, have you worn support stockings or tights?
6. In the last two weeks, have you had any itching in association with yourvaricose veins?
7. Do you have purple discolouration caused by tiny blood vessels in the skin, in association with your varicose veins?
8. Do you have a rash or eczema in the area of your ankle?
9. Do you have a skin ulcer associated with your varicose veins?
10. Does the appearance of your varicose veins cause you concern?
11. Does the appearance of your varicose veins influence your choice of clothing including tights?
12. During the last two weeks, have your varicose veins interfered with your work/housework or other daily activities?
13. During the last two weeks, have your varicose veins interfered with your leisure activities(including sport,hobbies and social life)?

4. SF36

SF-36 1

SF-36 Health survey

Instructions for completing the questionnaire: Please answer every question. Some questions may look like others, but each one is different. Please take the time to read and answer each question carefully by filling in the bubble that best represents your response.

Patient Name: _____
SSN#: _____ Date: _____
Person heling to complete this form: _____

1. In general, would you say your health is:

q Excellent
q Very good
q Good
q Fair
q Poor

2. Compared to one year ago, how would you rate your health in general now?

q Much better now than a year ago

q Somewhat better now than a year ago
q About the same as one year ago
q Somewhat worse now than one year ago
q Much worse now than one year ago

3. The following items are about activities you might do during a typical day. Does your health now limit you in these activities? If so, how much?

a. Vigorous activities, such as running, lifting heavy objects, participating in strenuous sports.
q Yes, limited a lot.
q Yes, limited a little.
q No, not limited at all.
b. Moderate activities, such as moving a table, pushing a vacuum cleaner, bowling, or playing golf?
q Yes, limited a lot.
q Yes, limited a little.
q No, not limited at all.
c. Lifting or carrying groceries.
q Yes, limited a lot.
q Yes, limited a little.
q No, not limited at all.
d. Climbing several flights of stairs.
q Yes, limited a lot.
q Yes, limited a little.
q No, not limited at all.
e. Climbing one flight of stairs.
q Yes, limited a lot.
q Yes, limited a little.
q No, not limited at all.
f. Bending, kneeling or stooping.
q Yes, limited a lot.
q Yes, limited a little.
q No, not limited at all.

SF-36 2

g. Walking more than one mile.
q Yes, limited a lot.
q Yes, limited a little.
q No, not limited at all.
h. Walking several blocks.
q Yes, limited a lot.
q Yes, limited a little.
q No, not limited at all.

i. Walking one block.
q Yes, limited a lot.
q Yes, limited a little.
q No, not limited at all.
j. Bathing or dressing yourself.
q Yes, limited a lot.
q Yes, limited a little.
q No, not limited at all.

4. During the past 4 weeks, have you had any of the following problems with your work or other regular daily activities as a result of your physical health?

a. Cut down the amount of time you spent on work or other activities?
c Yes c No
b. Accomplished less than you would like?
c Yes c No
c. Were limited in the kind of work or other activities
c Yes c No
d. Had difficulty performing the work or other activities (for example, it took extra time)
c Yes c No

5. During the past 4 weeks, have you had any of the following problems with your work or other regular daily activities as a result of any emotional problems (such as feeling depressed or anxious)?

a. Cut down the amount of time you spent on work or other activities?
c Yes c No
b. Accomplished less than you would like
c Yes c No
c. Didn't do work or other activities as carefully as usual
c Yes c No

6. During the past 4 weeks, to what extent has your physical health or emotional problems interfered with your normal social activities with family, friends, neighbors, or groups?

q Not at all
q Slightly
q Moderately
q Quite a bit
q Extremely

7. How much bodily pain have you had during the past 4 weeks?

q Not at all
q Slightly
q Moderately
q Quite a bit

q Extremely

SF-36 3

8. During the past 4 weeks, how much did pain interfere with your normal work (including both work outside the home and housework)?

q Not at all
q Slightly
q Moderately
q Quite a bit
q Extremely

9. These questions are about how you feel and how things have been with you during the past 4 weeks. For each question, please give the one answer that comes closest to the way you have been feeling. How much of the time during the past 4 weeks.

a. did you feel full of pep?
q All of the time
q Most of the time
q A good bit of the time
q Some of the time
q A little of the time
q None of the time
b. have you been a very nervous person?
q All of the time
q Most of the time
q A good bit of the time
q Some of the time
q A little of the time
q None of the time
c. have you felt so down in the dumps nothing could cheer you up?
q All of the time
q Most of the time
q A good bit of the time
q Some of the time
q A little of the time
q None of the time
d. have you felt calm and peaceful?
q All of the time
q Most of the time
q A good bit of the time
q Some of the time
q A little of the time
q None of the time

e. did you have a lot of energy?
q All of the time
q Most of the time
q A good bit of the time
q Some of the time
q A little of the time
q None of the time
f. have you felt downhearted and blue?
q All of the time
q Most of the time
q A good bit of the time
q Some of the time
q A little of the time
q None of the time

SF-36 4

g. did you feel worn out?
q All of the time
q Most of the time
q A good bit of the time
q Some of the time
q A little of the time
q None of the time
h. have you been a happy person?
q All of the time
q Most of the time
q A good bit of the time
q Some of the time
q A little of the time
q None of the time
i. did you feel tired?
q All of the time
q Most of the time
q A good bit of the time
q Some of the time
q A little of the time
q None of the time

10. During the past 4 weeks, how much of the time has your physical health or emotional problems interfered with your social activities (like visiting friends, relatives, etc.)?

q All of the time
q Most of the time
q Some of the time

q A little of the time
q None of the time

11. How TRUE or FALSE is each of the following statements for you?

a. I seem to get sick a little easier than other people
q Definitely true
q Mostly true
q Don't know
q Mostly false
q Definitely false
b. I am as healthy as anybody I know
q Definitely true
q Mostly true
q Don't know
q Mostly false
q Definitely false
c. I expect my health to get worse
q Definitely true
q Mostly true
q Don't know
q Mostly false
q Definitely false
d. My health is excellent
q Definitely true
q Mostly true
q Don't know
q Mostly false
q Definitely false

The clinical component from CEAP scores ranges from 0 to 6; Higher scores denote greater severity.

The VCSS consist of clinical variables, each ranging from 0(none) to 3 (severe). Thus, the VCSS ranged form 0 to 30; Higher scores denote greater severity of varicose veins.

The AVVSS assessment consisted of 13 clinical variables and the completion of a vein grid. Each question was given a weighted score. For each limb, the AVVSS produced a score ranging from 0 to 50; Higher scores meant greater severity of Varicose Veins.

The SF-36 is a multi-purpose, short-form health survey with only 36 questions. It yields an 8-scale profile of functional health and well-being scores as well as psychometrically-based physical and mental health summary measures and a preference-based health utility index. It is a generic measure, as opposed to one that targets a specific age, disease, or treatment group. Accordingly, the SF-36 has proven useful in surveys of general and specific populations, comparing the relative burden of diseases, and in differentiating the health benefits produced by a wide range of different treatments.

3. Operative details

The procedure was carried out by, or supervised by, a single consultant.

Patients were prepared with non alcoholic povidone-iodine and drapped with sterile disposable materials.

1% Lignocaine with Adrenaline was used to anaesthesize the groin and perform a Ilio-inguinal nerve block, according with the guidelines of Local Anaesthetic use [11] (Figure 2)

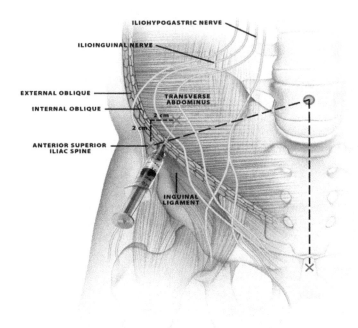

Figure 2.

The incision in the groin is placed medial to the Femoral pulse and 1 centimetre above the inguinal crease.

The dissection begins with the identification of the Long Saphenous Vein and the Sapheno-Femoral junction where the Long Saphenous Vein joins the Deep Femoral Vein. All tributaries of the Long Saphenous Vein are tied with 3.0 Vicryl sutures (Ethicon Inc Somerville, NJ). Smaller tributaries are dealt with Bipolar Diathermy. The proximal end of the Long Saphenous Vein is suture-ligated with 1.0 Vicryl and disconnected 0.5 cm flush from the Deep Femoral Vein.

Fascial layers are closed with interrupted 2.0 Vicryl sutures and the skin approximated with 2.0 Monocryl sutures (Ethicon Inc., Somerville, NJ).

Patients go back to the Day Unit where they are observed for 2 hours after their proedure and discharged from the Unit provided there are not complications.

3.1. Follow up

All patients who had Sapheno-Femoral junction Ligation and Disconnection(SFJLD) under Local Anaesthetic were reviewed in the Outpatient Department at 1,3 and 6 months postoperatively. At each of this times, the veins were examined clinically, marked and measured with the cartographer's wheel and the four questionnaires were repeated.

After a final assessment post- SFJLD, patients are listed for Multiple Stab Avulsions under Local Anaesthetic.

A three month Outpatient Department appointment is given to every patient for futher clinical assessment. In addition, all patients were contacted at the end of the study to assess the recurrence of Varicose Veins.

3.2. Statistics

The data collected were found to be parametric. The repeated measures analysis of variance test was used to compare continuous variables within the same groups of patients. Means and 95% confidence intervals were calculated for all variables. A p value of <0.05 was deemed significant

3.3. Results

There were 48 patients (15 men; mean age: 54 years; 95% CI: 29-79). Mean follow-up period after surgery was 43 (95% CI: 38-48) months. In all, 30 (91%) patients had immediate cosmetic and symptomatic improvement after surgery.

On follow-up, the volume of VV reduced significantly over the three postoperative time points when compared with preoperatively (112 [95% CI: 88-136] vs. 75 [95% CI: 55-97] vs. 65 [95% CI: 43-87] vs. 58 [95% CI: 31-86], $p = 0.001$) (Fig. 3).

Using the CEAP (Fig. 4), VCSS (Fig. 5), and AVVSS (Fig. 6) questionnaires, severity of VV improved postoperatively when compared with preoperatively ($p = 0.001$ for all three). Likewise, using the SF-36 questionnaire, significant improvements in quality of life were noted postoperatively (Fig. 7) ($p = 0.032$).

The results from the aforementioned analysis suggest that improvement in both the extent and severity of VV can occur to a maximum of 6 months after SFJLD under local anaesthetic. The second-stage procedure of multiple stab avulsions can therefore be performed to a maximum of 6 months after the index procedure without clinical deterioration.

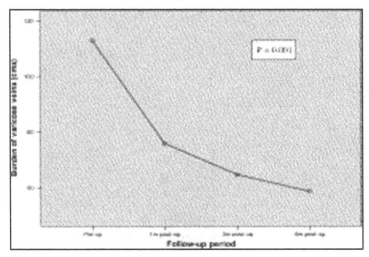

Figure 3. Follow-up of burden of varicose veins after surgery.

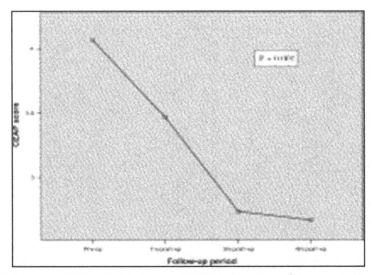

Figure 4. Follow-up of Clinical Etiology Anatomy Pathology scores after surgery.

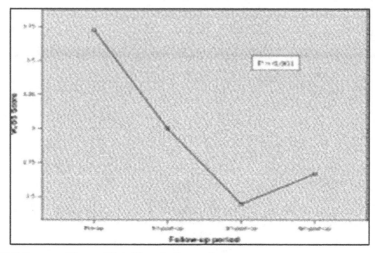

Figure 5. Follow-up of Venous Clinical Severity Scores after surgery.

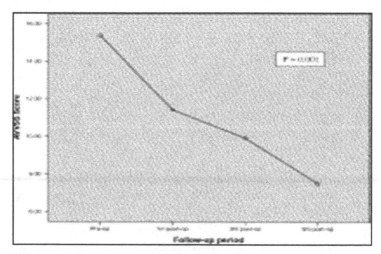

Figure 6. Follow-up of Aberdeen Varicose Vein Severity Scores after surgery.

On maximum follow-up, six (13%) patients had recurrent VV. Of these, two patients opted for redo surgery. This consisted of re-exploration of the groin and stripping of the long saphenous veins under a general anaesthetic.

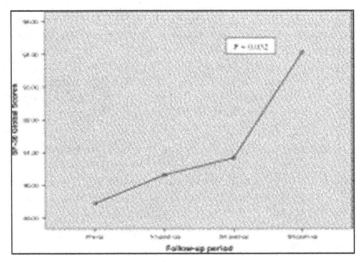

Figure 7. Follow-up of Short Form 36 scores after surgery.

4. Discussion

The results from present study suggest that SFJLD under local anaesthetic confers symptomatic and cosmetic improvement 1 month after the procedure. Improvements are sustained on early follow-up, thereby allowing multiple stab avulsions to be performed as a staged procedure within 6 months of the index procedure.

Currently, there is an increasing demand and need for VV surgery. Despite this demand, waiting lists are increasingly "controlled" and the funding is "regulated" by primary care trusts because VV are deemed to be a cosmetic disease without any life-threatening consequences. Ligation of the great saphenous vein at the SFJ, with or without stripping, is a long described method of VV surgery with varying successes [12, 13, 14]. We believe that SFJLD under a local anaesthetic, is a feasible procedure for VV disease, particularly for those with early disease. There are several advantages. Our method does not require a general anaesthetic and the procedure can be done as a day case without an in-patient stay. As such, surgery for VV can be done in peripheral cottage hospitals where specialized equipment and support from anaesthetic colleagues may be unavailable. The shift of work to peripheral hospitals reduces the demand and pressure on waiting list in larger central hospitals where general anaesthetic lists are being done.

The results obtained from the various VV questionnaires were reassuring. The procedure used in the present study resulted in significant cosmetic and functional improvement on short-term follow-up. We saw significant improvements with all three VV-specific questionnaires (CEAP, VCSS, and AVVSS questionnaire). Although the AVVSS questionnaire was initially designed to assess severity of varicosities in both lower limbs, we were still able to use it for unilateral assessment. The assessment was performed unilaterally in our series of patients because the total volume of local anaesthetic that was used for the procedure was often the limiting factor in surgery. Results from the SF-36 questionnaire have to be interpreted with caution. We noted significant improvements in quality of life up to 6 months postoperatively. The SF-36 is a global quality of life questionnaire, which may not be sensitive enough to detect improvements in quality of life as a direct consequence of VV surgery. However, to date, we are unaware of a more specific quality of life questionnaire, which has been designed for patients who underwent VV surgery.

There were several limitations to our study. First, the size of our patient population was small. We have been selective in the recruitment of patients for this study. Patients in our study had simple VV with minimal chronic venous changes; thus, they were patients who had early VV. We did not perform Duplex studies in any patients preoperatively. Certainly, the rates of early recurrent VV in our study are higher than conventional studies and this may be secondary to our failure to perform Duplex studies. This would have identified the anatomy of the long saphenous veins and potential perforators associated with it.

To further validate the study it may have been useful to have pre- and postoperative formal Duplex studies for comparison and to help explain disease recurrence. The reported rate of clinical recurrence ranges from 20 to 80% after a period between 5 and 20 years [15]. The average time between the first and the second surgical treatments is long ranging, from 6 to 20 years [16, 17].

As long-term data are lacking in our series, our recurrence rate of 13% at maximum 3 years follow-up may underestimate total disease recurrence. At 2 years follow-up, a recurrence rate of 16% was demonstrated by clinical and Duplex evaluation in a study by Coufinhal [18]

The rate of disease recurrence increases with time, probably because of progression of the disease. Kostas et al identified three main causes of disease recurrence [19]. The first was attributable to inadequate initial treatment and results in recurrence in 55-70% of cases. It arises either as a result of failure in identifying all incompetent veins or a failure in carrying out adequate primary treatment. The second group of causes arises from disease progression resulting in development of varices in previously normal veins and accounting for 20-25% of recurrences. The third cause of recurrence is neovascularization, in which varices arise in the track of previously stripped or ligated veins and account for 5-25% of recurrences. Dissection of the tributary vessels at the SFJ may contribute to our early rates of recurrence. Taking vessels back beyond the primary, or even the secondary tributaries, may be a cause of neovascularization in the groin. Duplex ultrasound surveillance has supported this finding [20].

5. Conclusion

SFJLD under local anaesthetic is a suitable procedure with early VV. Patients who undergo this procedure show improvement in cosmesis and function. However, on short-term follow-up, it appears to be associated with higher rates of recurrent VV when compared with conventional techniques.

Author details

Jesus Barandiaran, Thomas Hall, Naif El-Barghouti and Eugene Perry
Department of Surgery, Scarborough General Hospital, UK

6. References

[1] Rigby K A, Palfreyman S S J, Beverley C, Michaels J A. Surgery versus sclerotherapy for the treatment of varicose veins. Cochrane database reviews 2004, Issue 4. Art No.: CD004980.DOI: 10.1002/14651.CD004980.

[2] Wolf B, Brittenden J. Surgical treatment of varicose veins. JR Coll Sur Edin. 2001; 46: 154-158

[3] Callam M J. Epidemiology of varicose veins Br. J. Surg. 1994; 81: 168-173

[4] Bradbury A, Evans C, Allan P et all. What are the symptoms of varicose veins? Edinburgh vein study cross sectional population survey. BMJ. 1999; 6: 318-356

[5] Badri H., Bhattacharya V. A review of current treatment strategies for varicose veins. Recent Pat Cardiovasc Drug Disco. 2008; 3: 126-136

[6] Available at: www.NICE.org.uk/guidelines.

[7] Classification and grading of chronic venous disease in the lower limbs. A consensus statement. Ad Hoc Committee, American Venous Forum. *J Cardiovasc Surg (Torino)*. 1997;38:437–441

[8] Rutherford RB, Padberg FT, Comerota AJ, Kistner RL, Meissner MH, Moneta GL. Venous severity scoring: an adjunct to venous outcome assessments. J Vasc Surg. 2000;31:1307–1312

[9] Garratt AM, Macdonald LM, Ruta DA, Russell IT, Buckingham JK, Krukowski ZH. Towards measurements of outcomes for patients with varicose veins. Qual Health Care. 1993;2:5–10

[10] Ware JE, Kosinski M, Dewey JE. How to score version two of the SF-36 Health Survey. Lincoln, RI: Quality Metric Incorporated; 2000;

[11] British National Formulary. Available at: http://bnf.org/.

[12] Sarin S, Scurr JH, Coleridge Smith PD. Stripping of the long saphenous vein in the treatment of primary varicose veins. *Br J Surg*. 1994;81:1455–1458

[13] Rutgers PH, Kitslaar PJ. Randomized trial of stripping versus high ligation combined with sclerotherapy in the treatment of the incompetent greater saphenous vein. *Am J Surg*. 1994;168:311–315

[14] Hammarsten J, Pederson P, Cederlund CG, Campanello M. Long saphenous vein saving surgery for varicose veins: a long-term follow-up. *Eur J Vasc Surg*. 1990;4:361–364

[15] Eklof B, Juhan C. Recurrences of primary varicose veins. In: Eklof B, Gores E, Thulesius O, Berqvist O editor. Controversies in the Management of Venous Disorders. London, UK: Bitterworths; 1989;p. 220–233

[16] Darke S. The morphology of recurrent varicose veins. *Eur J Vasc Surg*. 1992;6:512–517

[17] Kostas T, Ioannou CV, Touloupakis E, Dastalaki E, Giannoukas AD, Tsetis D, et al. Recurrent varicose veins after surgery: a new appraisal of a common and complex problem in vascular surgery. *Eur J Vasc Endovasc Surg*. 2004;27:275–282

[18] Coufinhal JC. Récidive de varices après chirurgie: definition, épidémiologie, physiopathologie. In: Kieffer B, Bahnini A editor. Chirurgie des Veines des Members Infe`rieurs. Paris, France: AERCV; 1996;p. 227–238

[19] Kostas T, Ioannou CV, Touloupakis E, Dastalaki E, Giannoukas AD, Tsetis D, et al. Recurrent varicose veins after surgery: a new appraisal of a common and complex problem in vascular surgery. *Eur J Vasc Endovasc Surg*. 2004;27:275–282

[20] Van Rij AM, Jiang P, Solomon C, Christie RA, Hill GB. Recurrence after varicose vein surgery: a prospective long-term clinical study with duplex ultrasound scanning and air plethysmography. *J Vasc Surg*. 2003;38:935–943

The Role of Supervised Exercise Therapy in Peripheral Arterial Obstructive Disease

H.J.P. Fokkenrood, G.J. Lauret, M.R.M. Scheltinga,
H.J.M. Hendriks, R.A. de Bie and J.A.W. Teijink

Additional information is available at the end of the chapter

1. Introduction

Peripheral arterial occlusive disease (PAOD) commonly results from progressive narrowing or occlusion of arteries in the lower extremities mostly due to atherosclerosis. The atherosclerotic process of progressive narrowing and hardening of arteries can occur in each artery in the human body, however it mainly affects coronary, cerebral and peripheral arteries especially those in the lower extremities(1). The preferential sites of involvement of PAOD are the femoral and popliteal arteries in 80-90%, the tibial and peroneal arteries in 40-50% and in 30% the aorta and iliac arteries(2). The manifestation of PAOD ranges from no symptoms to tissue loss that may eventually requires amputation of an affected limb. The majority of patients with PAOD have asymptomatic or atypical disease (figure 1).

Total disease prevalence based on objective testing has been evaluated in several epidemiologic studies and ranges from 3% to 10% in adults, increasing to 15 to 20% in persons over 70 years. PAOD increases progressively with age, beginning after the age of 40(3). The relationship between PAOD prevalence and age was illustrated on data from the 1999–2000 National Health and Nutrition Examination Survey (NHANES), an ongoing cross-sectional survey of the civilian, non-institutionalized population of the United States. The prevalence of PAOD, defined as an ankle-brachial index (ABI) <0.90 in either leg, was 0.9% between the ages of 40-49, 2.5% between the ages of 50-59, 4.7% between the ages of 60-69, and 14.5% in ages 70 and older(3). These numbers indicate that PAOD affects more than 5 million adults in the United States, while international guidelines reveal some 27 million affected individuals in North America and Europe(1). The PARTNERS study (PAOD Awareness, Risk, and Treatment: New Resources for Survival) screened 6979 subjects for PAOD using the ABI (with PAOD defined as an ABI of ≤0.90 or a prior history of lower extremity revascularization)(4). Subjects were evaluated in primary care practices in the

United States if they were above 70 years of age or between 50–69 years when presenting with a risk factor for vascular disease (smoking, diabetes). PAOD was detected in 1865 patients (29% of the cohort). Classic claudication or symptomatic PAOD was present in only 5.5% of the newly diagnosed patients with PAOD. Some 12.6% of the patients with a prior diagnosis of PAOD had claudication. Other studies have evaluated symptomatic and asymptomatic PAOD patients in the same population. The ratio of the two is independent of age and is usually in the range of 1:3 to 1:4(1). It may be concluded that PAOD is still growing as a clinical problem due to the increasingly aged population in developed countries.

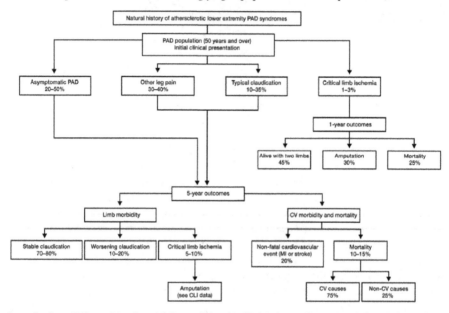

Legend to figure: PAD – peripheral arterial disease; CLI – critical limb ischemia; CV – cardiovascular; MI – myocardial infarction.

Figure 1. 5 years disease prognosis in claudicants (adapted from TASC II guidelines (1)).

2. Etiology of symptomatic PAOD (Intermittent Claudication)

50 – 80 % of PAOD patients are symptomatic and because of their complaints most of them will present themselves at a patient outdoor clinic. Symptomatic PAOD patients will have in 20-50% of the cases symptoms of typical intermittent claudication (IC, which means 'to limp') (figure 1). IC is defined as muscle discomfort in the lower limb reproducibly elicited by exercise and relieved by rest within 10 minutes(1).

Patients with IC have sufficient blood flow at rest and, therefore do not experience limb symptoms at rest. With exercise, occlusive or narrowing lesions in the arterial supply of the leg muscles limit the increase in blood flow resulting in a mismatch of oxygen supply and muscle metabolic demand that is associated with the symptom of claudication. This mismatch causes cramping or aching pain in the buttock, hip, thigh, calf or in rare occasions the foot, forcing the patient to pause. In rest, the oxygen debt can be redeemed and symptoms are relieved. In women, the incidence rates of IC are approximately 50% lower than in men(5). IC has an approximately 3% prevalence in the general population in patients aged 40 up to 6% in patients aged 60 years and increasing in older age(1).

Vascular origin - Major causes
Atherosclerosis
Thombosed aneurysm
Arterial injury
Arterial dissection
Atheroembolism
Thromboembolism
Thromboangiitis obliterans (Buerger's disease)
Vascular origin - Other causes
Aorto-iliac
Retroperitoneal fibrosis
Radiation fibrosis
Tumor
Takayasu's disease
Iliac
Fibromuscular dysplasia
Iliac endofibrosis (athletic injury)
Iliofemoral
Pseudoxanthoma elasticum
Popliteal
Popliteal entrapment
Adventitial cystic disease

Table 1. Etiology of lower extremity ischemia

Nerve root compression
Spinal stenosis
Hip / foot arthritis
Arthritic, inflammatory processes
Compartment syndrome
Venous claudication
Symptomatic Bakers cyste

Table 2. Common differential diagnoses of non – vascular origin.

Eventually any process that results in arterial stenosis or occlusion can cause symptoms of claudication, ischemic pain, or tissue loss but the vast majority of patients with claudication suffer from atherosclerosis. Aetiologies of lower extremity ischemia due to arterial stenosis or occlusion other than atherosclerosis are shown in table 1.

Arterial aneurysms can be the source of embolic debris leading to arterial obstruction resulting in symptoms of lower extremity ischemia. Popliteal entrapment syndrome can also present with IC and should be suspected in the young patient who presents with claudication but lacks atherosclerotic risk factors. In endurance athletes, especially cyclists, an even more unusual cause of claudication is due to repeated trauma (stretching or kinking) of the external iliac artery which can result in endofibrosis of the vessel(6).

Other diseases of non-vascular origin should also be considered in the differential diagnosis of leg pain (table 2). These include neurological, musculoskeletal and venous disorders. Neurological pain ("spinal claudication") is predominantly due to neurospinal (eg, disc disease, spinal stenosis, tumor) or neuropathic causes (eg, diabetes, alcohol abuse). Musculoskeletal pain derives from the bones, joints, ligaments, tendons, and fascial elements of the lower extremity. Clinical history taking and physical examination can help distinguish between some of the less common causes of these disorders, which is important to instate an effective treatment for a patient with IC complaints.

3. Prognostics and mortality

PAOD and IC are strong predictors for coinciding atherosclerotic disease and related mortality. The prevalence of cerebrovascular disease in patients with PAOD is about 25-50%(7). The 10-year mortality rate due to cardiovascular disease is 62% for men with PAOD compared to 17% in the population of men without PAOD. For women with PAOD the 10-year mortality rate is 33% compared to 12% without PAOD(8). In a subgroup of patients with severe and symptomatic PAOD a 15-fold increase in mortality rate was found(8).

For IC, a 5-year mortality rate of 19.2 % is described, of which 70% is due to cardiovascular causes. Non-fatal cardiovascular events (e.g. myocardial infarction, stroke) in patients with IC are found in 29% at 5 years of follow-up(5). Compared to patients with IC, subjects with asymptomatic PAOD appear to have the same increased risk of cardiovascular events and death(5). Nonetheless, for those afflicted, IC impacts negatively on walking ability and health-related quality of life (QoL)(9, 10).

4. General management of PAOD

PAOD comes with serious health risks. An overall strategy and basic treatment is well described in several international guidelines like the American College of Cardiology/ American Heart Association (ACC/AHA) and Trans-Atlantic Inter-Society Consensus on Management of Peripheral Arterial Disease (TASC II)(1, 11). Treatment of PAOD should consist of a multicomponent therapy of cardiovascular risk reduction (1) including lifestyle coaching (2) and symptomatic treatment (3). The first two components aim to prevent cardiovascular events (myocardial infarction, stroke) and related morbidity and mortality. The most important modifiable risk factors for atherosclerosis are smoking, hypertension, diabetes mellitus, hyperlipidemia and obesity(12). The third component is to improve QoL and realized with daily exercise supplemented with supervised exercise therapy (SET).

5. Smoking cessation

Smoking is a potent risk factor for symptomatic PAOD, with an important and consistent dose-response relationship(13). The prevalence of symptomatic PAOD was increased 2.3-fold in current smokers. Even in former smokers the prevalence was substantially increased by a factor of 2.6. Smoking cessation is associated with a decline in the incidence of IC. Results from the Edinburgh Artery Study found that the relative risk of IC was 3.7 in smokers compared with 3.0 in ex-smokers (who had discontinued smoking for less than 5 years)(1). In a meta-analysis of 12,603 smokers who had prior MI, CABG, angioplasty, or known coronary heart disease, the relative risk of mortality for quitters compared with those who continued to smoke was 0.64 (95% CI 0.58-0.71)(14). Observational studies have found that the risk of death, myocardial infarction and amputation is substantially greater, and lower extremity angioplasty and open surgical revascularization patency rates are lower in individuals with PAOD who continue to smoke than in those who stop smoking(15). Efforts to achieve smoking cessation are recommended for patients with lower extremity PAOD(13). A physician advice coupled with frequent follow-up achieves 1-year smoking cessation rates of approximately 5% compared with only 0.1% in individuals who try to quit smoking without a physician's intervention(16). In patients with PAOD, comprehensive smoking cessation programs that included individualized counseling and pharmacological support significantly increased the rate of smoking cessation at 6 months compared with verbal advice to quit smoking (21.3% versus 6.8%, p<0.02)(17). Therefore the focused update of the guideline for the management of smoking patients recommended that current smokers or former smokers should be asked about their status of tobacco use at every visit (Level of Evidence: A). Furthermore patients should be assisted with counseling and developing a plan for quitting that may include pharmacotherapy and/or referral to a smoking cessation program(15).

6. Hypertension

Hypertension is a major risk factor for PAOD. However, data evaluating whether antihypertensive therapy alters the progression of claudication are lacking. Nevertheless, international guidelines support the treatment of hypertension in patients with PAOD to reduce morbidity from cardiovascular and cerebrovascular disease. In this high-risk group the current recommendation is a goal of 140/90 mmHg, or even 130/80 mmHg if the patient also has diabetes or renal insufficiency. In PAOD, thiazides and ACE inhibitors should be considered as initial blood-pressure lowering drugs to reduce the risk of cardiovascular events. Beta-adrenergic blocking drugs have been discouraged in PAOD because of the possibility of worsening claudication symptoms. In a Cochrane review there was no supporting evidence that beta blockers adversely affect walking distance in people with IC(18). However, due to the lack of large published trials beta blockers should be used with caution but are not contraindicated in PAOD.

7. Diabetes mellitus

Diabetes increases the risk of PAOD approximately three- to four-fold, and the risk of claudication two-fold. Diabetes is also associated with peripheral neuropathy which may lead to an increased risk of foot ulcers and foot infections. In recent years, there has been much discussion about the optimal treatment strategy of type 2 diabetes mellitus, aggressive or standard glucose lowering therapy. In a meta-analysis, an intensive glucose lowering regime (glycated haemoglobin level below 6.0%) was compared to standard therapy (targeted a level of 7.0-7.9%) in type 2 diabetes mellitus. Overall, intensive therapy significantly reduced coronary events without a significant effect on events of stroke or all-cause mortality(19). However, aggressive control of blood glucose levels (glycated haemoglobin level below 6.0%) is not recommended. The long term results of intensive therapy described a significantly reduced nonfatal myocardial infarction risk but an increased all-cause mortality rate (hazard ratio 1.21; 95% C.I. 1.02-1.44) after 5-year related with aggressive glucose lowering(20). TASC II recommends moderate aggressive control of blood glucose levels with an A1C goal of <7.0% and as close to 6.0% as possible (but not below 6%)(1).

8. Hyperlipidemia

In case of hyperlipidemia, dietary modification should be the initial intervention to control abnormal lipid levels. A 2007 Cochrane meta-analysis of mostly older trials that specifically evaluated patients with lower limb atherosclerosis concluded that lipid-lowering therapy reduced disease progression (improvement in total walking distance (Mean Difference (MD) 152 m; 95% CI 32.11 to 271.88) and pain-free walking distance (WMD 89.76 m; 95% CI 30.05 to 149.47) but no significant impact on ankle brachial index (WMD 0.04; 95% CI -0.01 to 0.09)(21). It was concluded that lipid-lowering therapy is effective in reducing cardiovascular mortality and morbidity in people with PAOD. It may also improve local symptoms. Until further evidence on the relative effectiveness of different lipid-lowering agents is available, use of a statin in people with PAOD and a blood total cholesterol level ≥ 3.5 mmol/litre is indicated. One of the largest included studies in this Cochrane review, the Heart Protection Study demonstrated the benefits of cholesterol-lowering statin therapy in 6.748 patients with PAOD and 13.788 other high-risk participants, allocation to 40 mg simvastatin daily reduced the rate of the first major vascular events by about one-quarter, and that of peripheral vascular events by about one-sixth, with large absolute benefits seen in participants with PAOD because of their high vascular risk. Consequently, according to this study statin therapy should be considered for all patients with PAOD (all patients with total cholesterol level ≥ 3.5 mmol/L). This is in contrast to the older ACC/AHA guidelines as they recommended achieving an LDL cholesterol level <2.59 mmol/L (<100 mg/dL) in all patients with PAOD. In patients with PAOD and a history of other vascular disease (i.e., coronary heart disease and cerebrovascular disease) it is reasonable to lower LDL cholesterol levels to 1.81 mmol/L (70 mg/dL)(11). Statins should be the primary lipid-lowering agents to lower LDL cholesterol levels.

9. Blood homocysteine

Elevated homocysteine blood levels are associated with cardiovascular disease but it is uncertain whether this association is causal. Studies investigating the effects of folic acid supplementation on major vascular events in patients with peripheral arterial disease are lacking. However, long-term reductions in blood homocysteine levels with folic acid and vitamin B12 supplementation did not lead to a reduction of cardiovascular events and seems therefore not indicated according to a RCT including 12.064 survivors of myocardial infarction (22).

10. Antiplatelet therapy

Antiplatelet therapy reduces major vascular events (vascular death, nonfatal MI and nonfatal stroke) in patients with PAOD by 23%(23). Therefore, all symptomatic patients with or without a history of other cardiovascular disease should be prescribed antiplatelet therapy on the long term. Antiplatelet therapy is indicated to reduce the risk of MI, stroke and vascular death in individuals with symptomatic atherosclerotic lower extremity PAOD, including those with claudication. Aspirin is the antiplatelet agent of choice; clopidogrel may be used if aspirin cannot be tolerated or in the subgroup of patients with symptomatic PAOD(1). Unfortunately, adherence to cardiovascular medication is fairly low(24). Self-reported consistent use (reported on ≥2 consecutive follow-up surveys and then through death, withdrawal, or study end) of cardiovascular medication was analysed using the Duke Databank for Cardiovascular Disease in patients with coronary artery disease with or without heart failure. In 2002, consistent use was reported: for aspirin, 71%; beta-blockers, 46%; lipid-lowering therapy, 44%; aspirin and beta-blockers, 36%; and all three, 21%. For these reasons the assessment of medication compliance should be incorporated in the standard care for patients with PAOD, which is not the case in contemporary guidelines.

11. Pharmacological therapy for Intermittent Claudication

Pharmacologic treatment for relief of claudication symptoms typically involves other drugs than those used for risk reduction. Cilostazol is currently the most effective drug for IC(25). Approved by the FDA in 1999, the primary action of cilostazol is to inhibit phosphodiesterase type 3, which results in vasodilatation and inhibition of platelet aggregation, arterial thromboses and vascular smooth muscle proliferation. A three to six-month course of cilostazol is a possible first line pharmacotherapy for the relief of claudication symptoms. One study with 2702 patients having stable moderate to severe claudication were randomly assigned to cilostazol or placebo. Patients treated with 100 mg cilostazol twice daily for 12 to 24 weeks experienced significantly greater increases in maximal and pain-free walking distances (50% and 67%, versus 22% and 40%, respectively) compared to the placebo group(25). Naftidrofuryl can also be considered. In a meta-analysis, naftidrofuryl showed an clinically meaningful improvement in pain-free and maximum walking distance in patients with IC(26). It is a 5-hydroxytryptamine type 2 antagonist and may improve muscle metabolism and reduce erythrocyte and platelet aggregation. Approval of cilostazol or naftidrofuryl for IC is however limited to certain countries.

Other treatments are described such as the use of pentoxifylline (Trental). Pentotoxifylline is a rheologic modifier approved by the FDA for the symptomatic relief of claudication. Its mechanism of action includes an increase in red blood cell deformity wheras it decreases fibrinogen concentration, platelet adhesiveness, and whole-blood viscosity. The available data indicate that the benefit of pentoxifylline is marginal and not well established(11).

Ginkgo biloba has been studied in patients with claudication with modest success. The mechanism by which ginkgo may work in this disorder is unclear, but may involve a number of activities including an antioxidant effect, inhibition of vascular injury, and antithrombotic effects. In a meta-analysis of 11 trials, patients who received ginkgo biloba extract had no significant differences in initial claudication distance. However, a trend toward improvement in the absolute claudication distance was observed. With the treadmill distances standardized between the protocols, a mean difference of 3.57 (95% CI -0.10-4.19) was found that corresponded to about 200 feet (64 meters), but the difference was not significant(27). The TASC guidelines concluded that no effect was proven(1). Several studies have evaluated the role of Vitamin E, chelation therapy, omega-3 fatty acids and estrogen therapies in the treatment of claudication. However, none of these therapies appeared effective(1).

12. Exercise therapy

Exercise therapy is the first suggested therapy for patients with IC. In 1898 the German neurologist Wilhelm Erb described successful results of exercise therapy for a patient with IC(28). The first randomised clinical trial (RCT) was performed by Larsen en Lassen in 1966(29). In this study, 7 patients treated with exercise therapy were compared with a control group of 7 patients who were given 'medical treatment' in the form of lactose tablets. For the group treated with exercise, a significant increase in maximum walking time was observed whereas the patients in the control group did not improve.

Nowadays, exercise therapy for patients with IC is extensively studied. In a Cochrane review by Watson et al. exercise therapy was compared with usual care or placebo regarding data of functional capacity outcome measurements(30). A total of twenty-two trials met the inclusion criteria involving a total of 1200 participants. Compared to placebo and usual care, exercise therapy significantly improved maximal walking time with a mean difference of 5.12 minutes (95% confidence interval 4.51 – 5.72) and an improved maximum walking distance of 113.2 metres (range 95.0 to 131.4). Exercise therapy also showed a positive effect on the reduction of cardiovascular risk factors including hypercholesterolemia, hypertension, and diabetes mellitus.

The most common exercise therapy prescription consists of a single oral advice, usually without supervision or follow-up. The adherence of patients given an oral exercise advice appears to be low. Comorbidity, lack of (specific) advice, fear, and lack of discipline and supervision are barriers to actually perform regular walking exercise(31). For these reasons the importance of supervision was recognised.

13. Supervised exercise therapy vs usual care (exercise therapy)

Supervised exercise therapy (SET) entails adequate coaching by a physical therapist (PT) or an other exercise specialist (e.g. exercise physiologist, exercise therapist, specialised cardiovascular nurse) and aims to increase maximal walking distance, physical activity and health-related QoL. The most effective programs employ treadmill walking of sufficient intensity to cause claudication symptoms. Exercise is continued till near maximum pain, followed by rest, and then a next cycle of exercise is started over the course of a 30–60 minute session. During the exercise session, treadmill exercise is performed at a speed and grade that will induce claudication symptoms. The patient should stop walking when claudication pain is considered moderate (a less optimal training response will occur when the patient stops at the onset of claudication). Exercise sessions are typically conducted three times a week for 3 months. A Cochrane review by Bendermacher et al. compared SET with non-supervised exercise programmes for patients with IC(32). SET showed statistically significant and clinically relevant differences in improvement of maximal walking distance compared with non-supervised exercise therapy regimens, with an overall effect size of 0.58 (95% confidence interval 0.31 to 0.85) at three months. This translates into an improvement of approximately 150 meters of maximum walking distance in favour of the supervised group. However, additional studies on QoL are needed to definitely demonstrate clinical effectiveness.

Another systematic meta-analysis comparing supervised to unsupervised exercise therapy showed a weighted mean difference in Pain Free Walking Distance (PWD) and Absolute Walking Distance (AWD) of 143.8 meters (95% CI; 5.8e281.8) and 250.4 meters (95% CI; 192.4-308.5), respectively. The authors concluded that SET increased the PWD and AWD more than standard care(33). In a recent randomized controlled trial, three groups were compared: usual care (walk advice), home-based exercise and supervised exercise(34). Claudication Onset Time (COT) and Peak Walking Time (PWT) were compared after 3 months. A significant improvement in COT and PWT were obtained in the exercise groups, but not in the usual care group (change after 3 months (sec): usual care; COT -16s, PWT -10s; home-based; COT 134s, PWT 124s; supervised; COT 165s, PWT 215s).

14. Supervised exercise therapy vs endovascular revascularisation

A recent systematic review compared (S)ET with percutaneous transluminal angioplasty (PTA) in patients with intermittent claudication (IC) to obtain the best estimates of their relative effectiveness(35). Eleven studies (reporting data on eight randomized clinical trials) met the inclusion criteria. One trial included patients with isolated aortoiliac artery obstruction(36). In this MIMIC trial, patients were randomised to receive either PTA or no PTA against a background of SET and best medical therapy. The maximum walking distance was 75% greater in the PTA group (95%; CI 2-202) at 6 months and 78% greater in the PTA group (95%; CI 0-216) (p=0.05) at 24 months. No benefits were found for health-related QoL. Unfortunately this trial did not evaluate results of SET alone versus PTA alone, so there is no evidence that angioplasty alone would produce similar results.

In the review of Frans et al. three trials were included, which studied SET and PTA in femoropopliteal artery obstructions. In summary, SET with additional PTA gave the best improvement in Maximal Walking Distance (MWD), Initial Claudication Distance (ICD) and Ankle Brachial Index (ABI)(35). Changes in MWD, ICD and ABI between PTA alone and SET alone were equivocal, either comparable or in favour of PTA. QoL improved significantly during follow-up compared with baseline of all treatments, without differences between both groups.

The systematic review additionally included five trials that studied combined lesions(35). In summary, PTA plus SET compared with PTA alone demonstrated an improvement in MWD. The two trials evaluating SET versus PTA had inconsistent results: one showed a benefit in terms of MWD and ICD after SET. The other trial demonstrated equal benefit in both groups. QoL data was assessed by seven different instruments with equivalent results. In conclusion there is not yet a well defined consensus for tailoring the optimal treatment for lesions at different anatomical locations. International guidelines (TASC II) still suggests to perform revascularisation when proximal lesions are suspected instead of prescribing SET and medical therapy. Unfortunately these guidelines may seem outdated. Results described above one could conclude that, in general, the effectiveness of PTA and SET was equivalent, although PTA plus SET improved walking distance and some domains of QoL scales compared with SET or PTA alone(35). Evidence to use a combination of PTA and SET for patients with IC complaints is still inconclusive. Moreover, cost-effectiveness data is still missing.

In the United States, another large multicenter RCT was conducted(37). In this so called CLEVER trial, the researchers aimed to find the optimal treatment strategy for IC with endpoints being maximal walking duration and health-related QoL. They randomly assigned 111 patients with aortoiliac peripheral artery disease to receive 1 of 3 treatments: optimal medical care (OMC), OMC plus supervised exercise (SE), or OMC plus stent revascularization (ST). At the 6-month follow-up, the change in peak walking time (the primary end point) was greatest for SE, intermediate for ST, and least with OMC (mean change versus baseline, 5.8±4.6, 3.7±4.9, and 1.2±2.6 minutes, respectively; P<0.001 for the comparison of SE versus OMC, P<0.02 for ST versus OMC, and P<0.04 for SE versus ST). QoL improved with both SE and ST compared with OMC, for most scales, the extent of improvement was greater with ST than SE. The authors concluded that SE results in superior treadmill walking performance than ST, even for those with aortoiliac peripheral artery disease(37). The contrast between better walking performance for SE and better patient-reported quality of life for ST warrants further follow up.

In conclusion, combining results of both studies, one could suggest that all patients with symptomatic PAOD should receive SET first as part of the initial treatment regimen, even patients with proximal lesions. In case of failing (patient dissatisfaction, disappointing results) an additional PTA could be suggested. However this treatment advice is based on moderate-level evidence, therefore results of two new trials have to be awaited (see section "future perspectives").

15. Supervised exercise therapy versus surgical reconstruction

Only one RCT compared SET to surgical reconstruction(38). This study reported the initial evaluation of treatment efficiency in 75 patients with IC who were randomized to three treatment groups: 1) reconstructive surgery, 2) reconstructive surgery with subsequent physical training, and 3) physical training alone. The walking performance was improved in all three groups at follow-up, 13±0.5 months after randomization. Surgery was most effective, but the addition of training to surgery improved the symptom-free walking distance even further. However, no significant difference was found. Moreover, a higher complication rate and 3 deaths were observed in the surgical groups while no complications occurred in the trained group. Furthermore, the methodological quality of this trial could be questioned.

16. Long term effects of supervised exercise therapy

Few studies consider the long-term (>12 months) effects of SET. Gardner et al. tried to determine whether improvements in physical function after 6 months of SET could be sustained over a subsequent 12-months in older patients with IC(39). They concluded that improvements in maximum walking distance and physical activity level, after 6 months of exercise training, were prolonged for an additional 12 months period using a less intense exercise maintenance program. Ratliff et al. reported a 3-year follow-up of 212 patients with IC who initially were treated with SET with an exercise programme of two sessions a week for 10 weeks(40). Their results show that the maximum walking distance observed at 12 weeks was still present at three years. Based on this limited experience, it appears that SET may have long term benefits for patients with IC.

17. Supervised exercise therapy in hospital or community based setting

An outpatient hospital setting was offered in the majority of all reviewed studies on SET. This approach may seem appropriate in trials but is associated with several limitations in daily clinical practise. First, the capacity of an exercise therapy program in an outpatient clinic is limited and not sufficient to provide SET for all patients with IC. Second, attending a hospital 3 times a week leads to a considerable transportation fee and is time-consuming for an individual patient. For this reason, implementation of a community-based SET program was instigated(41). The first results of a cohort study of patients treated with community-based SET resulted in a highly statistically significant improvement in maximum walking distance (on a treadmill) after 3 and 6 months(42). The authors concluded that comparison of these results with historical studies on hospital-based SET should be done with caution due to the variability in the prescribed exercise regimens and used treadmill walking tests. However, SET in a community-based setting seemed to be at least as efficacious as programs that are provided in a clinical setting but with a higher capacity.

18. Cost effectiveness of SET

In a multicenter RCT 'ExitPAD' trial, Nicolaï et al. compared exercise therapy in the form of a 'go home and walk' advice (WA) with community-based SET for patients with IC(43). The data from this ExitPAD trial were also used to assess the cost-effectiveness of SET versus WA. For community-based SET, the incremental cost-effectiveness ratio for cost per QALY was €28,693. The Health Council of the Netherlands has determined that a QALY € 40,000 may cost if the burden of disease for symptomatic PAOD is stated at a value of 0.5. At a willingness-to-pay threshold of this €40,000 SET seemed a cost-effective therapeutic option for patients with PAOD. In another randomized cost-effectiveness analysis SET was compared with endovascular revascularization (angioplasty with or without stenting)(44). This study was unfortunately underpowered so no significant difference was obtained. Endovascular revascularization leaded to a non-significant increase of 0.01 in QALYs (CI - 0.05 to 0.07). However a significant difference was demonstrated with respect to treatment costs. The costs for endovascular revascularization were significantly higher with a mean difference of € 2,318 per patient. In conclusion, endovascular revascularization was found cost effective if society would be willing to pay € 231,800 per QALY. This amount is far above the threshold of € 40,000. Therefore endovascular revascularization seems not cost effective compared with SET.

Over the last decades, no international randomized cost-effectiveness analyses or health economic models were carried out to configure satisfying treatment strategies or guidelines. This while scientific evidence on the effectiveness of SET compared to endovascular revascularization has grown. Furthermore, the costs of endovascular revascularization will increase significantly as a result of technological innovations. SET seems the most cost-effective treatment for symptomatic PAOD certainly if potential positive effects due to lifestyle changes on other vascular diseases (such as heart failure, myocardial infarction, stroke) and reduction of risk factors (such as hypertension, diabetes mellitus, and hyperlipidaemia) are taken into count. Further research into the extent of cost effectiveness is an urgent need for policy choices in modern health care (see section future perspectives)(45).

19. Future perspectives

Although SET is considered the best evidence based therapy for all patients with IC, general practitioners, vascular surgeons or vascular specialists do not always have the disposal of (community-based) physical or exercise therapists (PTs) with specific knowledge of IC or exercise training. Also, not all PT's have sufficient experience with this specific patient category. Patients suffer from a variety of comorbidities and modifiable lifestyle factors, potentially generating suboptimal results. Unfortunately, too many examples of PT's treating patients with IC with massage and other alternative, non evidence based treatments exist.

In an ideal situation, all patients with symptomatic PAOD should receive an evidence based standardised form of SET by an exercise specialist. Due to lack of capacity, hospital-based exercise therapy should be reserved for cases with severe (cardiac) comorbidity. For this reason the ClaudicatioNet concept was launched in the Netherlands in January 2011. ClaudicatioNet is a concept representing an integrated care network between PTs, vascular surgeons and general practitioners. ClaudicatioNet aims to implement nationwide coverage of regional networks providing transparent, synergistic and multidisciplinary care according the guidelines of cardiovascular risk management and SET.

Two Dutch multicenter RCT's are including patients to evaluate the effectiveness and cost-effectiveness of SET. The ERASE-trial compares SET with a PTA complementary to SET. The optimal treatment strategy for IC due to an iliac artery obstruction will be determined in the SUPER-trial. The SUPER-trial compares the (cost-) effectiveness of initial PTA versus initial SET in patients with disabling IC due to an iliac artery obstruction. Results have to be awaited.

Although there is little evidence yet, SET could also be effective for patients with critical limb ischemia as an adjuvant to a revascularisation procedure. Badger et al. evaluated the efficacy of an exercise program following arterial bypass surgery for short distance IC or critical ischemia(46). SET resulted for this group in an increased maximum walking distance of 175% compared to 4% for the group with usual care. These studies indicate that SET is a useful adjunct after a PTA or lower limb bypass surgery. In the Netherlands the PEARL study is designed to confirm the clinical effectiveness of SET after a vascular intervention for the subgroup of patients with critical limb ischemia.

Author details

H.J.P. Fokkenrood[1,2], G.J. Lauret[1,2], M.R.M. Scheltinga[3],
H.J.M. Hendriks[2], R.A. de Bie[2] and J.A.W. Teijink[1,2]
[1]Department of Vascular Surgery, Catharina Hospital, Eindhoven, The Netherlands
[2]CAPHRI Research School, Department of Epidemiology, Maastricht University, The Netherlands
[3]Department of Vascular Surgery, Maxima Medical Centre, Veldhoven, The Netherlands

20. References

[1] Norgren L, Hiatt WR, Dormandy JA, Nehler MR, Harris KA, Fowkes FG. Inter-Society Consensus for the Management of Peripheral Arterial Disease (TASC II). J Vasc Surg. [Consensus Development Conference]. 2007 Jan;45 Suppl S:S5-67.

[2]   Fauci. Harrison's principles of internal medicine. 2 ed. New York: McGraw-Hill; 1998.

[3]   Selvin E, Erlinger TP. Prevalence of and risk factors for peripheral arterial disease in the United States: results from the National Health and Nutrition Examination Survey, 1999-2000. Circulation. [Research Support, U.S. Gov't, P.H.S.]. 2004 Aug 10;110(6):738-43.

[4]   Hirsch AT, Criqui MH, Treat-Jacobson D, Regensteiner JG, Creager MA, Olin JW, et al. Peripheral arterial disease detection, awareness, and treatment in primary care. Jama. [Multicenter Study Research Support, Non-U.S. Gov't Research Support, U.S. Gov't, P.H.S.]. 2001 Sep 19;286(11):1317-24.

[5]   Leng GC, Lee AJ, Fowkes FG, Whiteman M, Dunbar J, Housley E, et al. Incidence, natural history and cardiovascular events in symptomatic and asymptomatic peripheral arterial disease in the general population. Int J Epidemiol. [Research Support, Non-U.S. Gov't]. 1996 Dec;25(6):1172-81.

[6]   Schep G, Bender MH, van de Tempel G, Wijn PF, de Vries WR, Eikelboom BC. Detection and treatment of claudication due to functional iliac obstruction in top endurance athletes: a prospective study. Lancet. [Research Support, Non-U.S. Gov't]. 2002 Feb 9;359(9305):466-73.

[7]   Criqui MH. Systemic atherosclerosis risk and the mandate for intervention in atherosclerotic peripheral arterial disease. Am J Cardiol. [Review]. 2001 Oct 11;88(7B):43J-7J.

[8]   Criqui MH, Langer RD, Fronek A, Feigelson HS, Klauber MR, McCann TJ, et al. Mortality over a period of 10 years in patients with peripheral arterial disease. N Engl J Med. [Research Support, U.S. Gov't, P.H.S.]. 1992 Feb 6;326(6):381-6.

[9]   Regensteiner JG, Hiatt WR, Coll JR, Criqui MH, Treat-Jacobson D, McDermott MM, et al. The impact of peripheral arterial disease on health-related quality of life in the Peripheral Arterial Disease Awareness, Risk, and Treatment: New Resources for Survival (PARTNERS) Program. Vasc Med. [Comparative Study Multicenter Study Research Support, Non-U.S. Gov't]. 2008 Feb;13(1):15-24.

[10] Dumville JC, Lee AJ, Smith FB, Fowkes FG. The health-related quality of life of people with peripheral arterial disease in the community: the Edinburgh Artery Study. Br J Gen Pract. [Research Support, Non-U.S. Gov't]. 2004 Nov;54(508):826-31.

[11] Hirsch AT, Haskal ZJ, Hertzer NR, Bakal CW, Creager MA, Halperin JL, et al. ACC/AHA 2005 Practice Guidelines for the management of patients with peripheral arterial disease (lower extremity, renal, mesenteric, and abdominal aortic): a collaborative report from the American Association for Vascular Surgery/Society for Vascular Surgery, Society for Cardiovascular Angiography and Interventions, Society for Vascular Medicine and Biology, Society of Interventional Radiology, and the ACC/AHA Task Force on Practice Guidelines (Writing Committee to Develop Guidelines for the Management of Patients With Peripheral Arterial Disease): endorsed by the American Association of Cardiovascular and Pulmonary Rehabilitation; National Heart, Lung, and Blood Institute; Society for Vascular Nursing; TransAtlantic Inter-Society Consensus; and Vascular Disease Foundation. Circulation. [Practice Guideline Review]. 2006 Mar 21;113(11):e463-654.

[12] Dormandy J, Heeck L, Vig S. Predictors of early disease in the lower limbs. Semin Vasc Surg. [Review]. 1999 Jun;12(2):109-17.

[13] Willigendael EM, Teijink JA, Bartelink ML, Kuiken BW, Boiten J, Moll FL, et al. Influence of smoking on incidence and prevalence of peripheral arterial disease. J Vasc Surg. [Review]. 2004 Dec;40(6):1158-65.

[14] Critchley JA, Capewell S. Mortality risk reduction associated with smoking cessation in patients with coronary heart disease: a systematic review. Jama. [Research Support, Non-U.S. Gov't Review]. 2003 Jul 2;290(1):86-97.

[15] Rooke TW, Hirsch AT, Misra S, Sidawy AN, Beckman JA, Findeiss LK, et al. 2011 ACCF/AHA focused update of the guideline for the management of patients with peripheral artery disease (updating the 2005 guideline): a report of the American College of Cardiology Foundation/American Heart Association Task Force on Practice Guidelines: developed in collaboration with the Society for Cardiovascular Angiography and Interventions, Society of Interventional Radiology, Society for Vascular Medicine, and Society for Vascular Surgery. J Vasc Surg. [Practice Guideline Review]. 2011 Nov;54(5):e32-58.

[16] Law M, Tang JL. An analysis of the effectiveness of interventions intended to help people stop smoking. Arch Intern Med. [Research Support, Non-U.S. Gov't Review]. 1995 Oct 9;155(18):1933-41.

[17] Hennrikus D, Joseph AM, Lando HA, Duval S, Ukestad L, Kodl M, et al. Effectiveness of a smoking cessation program for peripheral artery disease patients: a randomized controlled trial. J Am Coll Cardiol. [Multicenter Study Randomized Controlled Trial Research Support, Non-U.S. Gov't]. 2010 Dec 14;56(25):2105-12.

[18] Paravastu SC, Mendonca D, Da Silva A. Beta blockers for peripheral arterial disease. Cochrane Database Syst Rev. [Meta-Analysis Review]. 2008(4):CD005508.

[19] Ray KK, Seshasai SR, Wijesuriya S, Sivakumaran R, Nethercott S, Preiss D, et al. Effect of intensive control of glucose on cardiovascular outcomes and death in patients with diabetes mellitus: a meta-analysis of randomised controlled trials. Lancet. [Meta-Analysis Research Support, Non-U.S. Gov't]. 2009 May 23;373(9677):1765-72.

[20] Gerstein HC, Miller ME, Genuth S, Ismail-Beigi F, Buse JB, Goff DC, Jr., et al. Long-term effects of intensive glucose lowering on cardiovascular outcomes. N Engl J Med. [Multicenter Study Randomized Controlled Trial Research Support, N.I.H., Extramural Research Support, U.S. Gov't, P.H.S.]. 2011 Mar 3;364(9):818-28.

[21] Aung PP, Maxwell HG, Jepson RG, Price JF, Leng GC. Lipid-lowering for peripheral arterial disease of the lower limb. Cochrane Database Syst Rev. [Meta-Analysis Review]. 2007(4):CD000123.

[22] Armitage JM, Bowman L, Clarke RJ, Wallendszus K, Bulbulia R, Rahimi K, et al. Effects of homocysteine-lowering with folic acid plus vitamin B12 vs placebo on mortality and major morbidity in myocardial infarction survivors: a randomized trial. Jama. [Multicenter Study Randomized Controlled Trial Research Support, Non-U.S. Gov't]. 2010 Jun 23;303(24):2486-94.

[23] Collaborative meta-analysis of randomised trials of antiplatelet therapy for prevention of death, myocardial infarction, and stroke in high risk patients. Bmj. [Meta-Analysis Research Support, Non-U.S. Gov't]. 2002 Jan 12;324(7329):71-86.

[24] Newby LK, LaPointe NM, Chen AY, Kramer JM, Hammill BG, DeLong ER, et al. Long-term adherence to evidence-based secondary prevention therapies in coronary artery disease. Circulation. [Research Support, U.S. Gov't, P.H.S.]. 2006 Jan 17;113(2):203-12.

[25] Thompson PD, Zimet R, Forbes WP, Zhang P. Meta-analysis of results from eight randomized, placebo-controlled trials on the effect of cilostazol on patients with intermittent claudication. Am J Cardiol. [Comparative Study Meta-Analysis Research Support, Non-U.S. Gov't]. 2002 Dec 15;90(12):1314-9.

[26] De Backer T, Vander Stichele R, Lehert P, Van Bortel L. Naftidrofuryl for intermittent claudication: meta-analysis based on individual patient data. Bmj. [Meta-Analysis Research Support, Non-U.S. Gov't Review]. 2009;338:b603.

[27] Nicolai SP, Kruidenier LM, Bendermacher BL, Prins MH, Teijink JA. Ginkgo biloba for intermittent claudication. Cochrane Database Syst Rev. [Meta-Analysis Review]. 2009(2):CD006888.

[28] Erb W. About intermittent walking and nerve disturbances due to vascular disease [Uber das "intermitterende Hinken" und adere nervose Storungen in Folge von Gefasserkrankungen] Deutsch Z Nervenheilk. 1898;13:1–76.

[29] Larsen OA, Lassen NA. Effect of daily muscular exercise in patients with intermittent claudication. Lancet. [Clinical Trial Randomized Controlled Trial]. 1966 Nov 19;2(7473):1093-6.

[30] Watson L, Ellis B, Leng GC. Exercise for intermittent claudication. Cochrane Database Syst Rev. [Meta-Analysis Review]. 2008(4):CD000990.

[31] Bartelink ML, Stoffers HE, Biesheuvel CJ, Hoes AW. Walking exercise in patients with intermittent claudication. Experience in routine clinical practice. Br J Gen Pract. [Research Support, Non-U.S. Gov't]. 2004 Mar;54(500):196-200.

[32] Bendermacher BL, Willigendael EM, Teijink JA, Prins MH. Supervised exercise therapy versus non-supervised exercise therapy for intermittent claudication. Cochrane Database Syst Rev. [Meta-Analysis Review]. 2006(2):CD005263.

[33] Wind J, Koelemay MJ. Exercise therapy and the additional effect of supervision on exercise therapy in patients with intermittent claudication. Systematic review of randomised controlled trials. Eur J Vasc Endovasc Surg. [Meta-Analysis Review]. 2007 Jul;34(1):1-9.

[34] Gardner AW, Parker DE, Montgomery PS, Scott KJ, Blevins SM. Efficacy of quantified home-based exercise and supervised exercise in patients with intermittent claudication: a randomized controlled trial. Circulation. [Comparative Study Randomized Controlled Trial Research Support, N.I.H., Extramural Research Support, Non-U.S. Gov't]. 2011 Feb 8;123(5):491-8.

[35] Frans FA, Bipat S, Reekers JA, Legemate DA, Koelemay MJ. Systematic review of exercise training or percutaneous transluminal angioplasty for intermittent claudication. Br J Surg. [Review]. 2012 Jan;99(1):16-28.

[36] Greenhalgh RM, Belch JJ, Brown LC, Gaines PA, Gao L, Reise JA, et al. The adjuvant benefit of angioplasty in patients with mild to moderate intermittent claudication (MIMIC) managed by supervised exercise, smoking cessation advice and best medical therapy: results from two randomised trials for stenotic femoropopliteal and aortoiliac arterial disease. Eur J Vasc Endovasc Surg. [Comparative Study Multicenter Study Randomized Controlled Trial Research Support, Non-U.S. Gov't]. 2008 Dec;36(6):680-8.

[37] Murphy TP, Cutlip DE, Regensteiner JG, Mohler ER, Cohen DJ, Reynolds MR, et al. Supervised exercise versus primary stenting for claudication resulting from aortoiliac peripheral artery disease: six-month outcomes from the claudication: exercise versus endoluminal revascularization (CLEVER) study. Circulation. [Comparative Study Multicenter Study Randomized Controlled Trial Research Support, N.I.H., Extramural Research Support, Non-U.S. Gov't]. 2012 Jan 3;125(1):130-9.

[38] Lundgren F, Dahllof AG, Lundholm K, Schersten T, Volkmann R. Intermittent claudication--surgical reconstruction or physical training? A prospective randomized trial of treatment efficiency. Ann Surg. [Clinical Trial Comparative Study Randomized Controlled Trial]. 1989 Mar;209(3):346-55.

[39] Gardner AW, Katzel LI, Sorkin JD, Goldberg AP. Effects of long-term exercise rehabilitation on claudication distances in patients with peripheral arterial disease: a randomized controlled trial. J Cardiopulm Rehabil. [Clinical Trial Randomized Controlled Trial Research Support, U.S. Gov't, Non-P.H.S. Research Support, U.S. Gov't, P.H.S.]. 2002 May-Jun;22(3):192-8.

[40] Ratliff DA, Puttick M, Libertiny G, Hicks RC, Earby LE, Richards T. Supervised exercise training for intermittent claudication: lasting benefit at three years. Eur J Vasc Endovasc Surg. 2007 Sep;34(3):322-6.

[41] Willigendael EM, Bendermacher BL, van der Berg C, Welten RJ, Prins MH, Bie de RA, et al. The development and implementation of a regional network of physiotherapists for exercise therapy in patients with peripheral arterial disease, a preliminary report. BMC Health Serv Res. 2005;5:49.

[42] Bendermacher BL, Willigendael EM, Nicolai SP, Kruidenier LM, Welten RJ, Hendriks E, et al. Supervised exercise therapy for intermittent claudication in a community-based setting is as effective as clinic-based. J Vasc Surg. [Clinical Trial Comparative Study Multicenter Study]. 2007 Jun;45(6):1192-6.

[43] van Asselt AD, Nicolai SP, Joore MA, Prins MH, Teijink JA. Cost-effectiveness of exercise therapy in patients with intermittent claudication: supervised exercise therapy versus a 'go home and walk' advice. Eur J Vasc Endovasc Surg. [Randomized Controlled Trial Research Support, Non-U.S. Gov't]. 2011 Jan;41(1):97-103.

[44] Spronk S, Bosch JL, den Hoed PT, Veen HF, Pattynama PM, Hunink MG. Cost-effectiveness of endovascular revascularization compared to supervised hospital-based exercise training in patients with intermittent claudication: a randomized controlled trial. J Vasc Surg. [Comparative Study Randomized Controlled Trial]. 2008 Dec;48(6):1472-80.

[45] Lauret GJ, van Dalen DC, Willigendael EM, Hendriks EJ, de Bie RA, Spronk S, et al. Supervised exercise therapy for intermittent claudication: current status and future perspectives. Vascular. 2012 Feb;20(1):12-9.

[46] Badger SA, Soong CV, O'Donnell ME, Boreham CA, McGuigan KE. Benefits of a supervised exercise program after lower limb bypass surgery. Vasc Endovascular Surg. [Randomized Controlled Trial]. 2007 Feb-Mar;41(1):27-32.

Chapter 6

Iatrogenic Pseudoaneurysms

Charles P.E. Milne, Regent Lee and Ashok I. Handa

Additional information is available at the end of the chapter

1. Introduction

A pseudoaneurysm refers to a defect in an arterial wall, which allows communication of arterial blood with the adjacent extra-luminal space. Blood extravasates out of the artery, but is contained by surrounding soft tissue and compressed thrombus which form a cavity or sac.[1] There is often a narrow tract stemming from the arterial wall to the pseudoaneurysm sac, termed the 'neck'. A pseudoaneurysm is distinct from a 'true' aneurysm, which results from dilation of all layers of the arterial wall.

Pseudoaneurysms are typically the result of traumatic arterial injury. With the increasing utilisation of percutaneous arterial interventions worldwide, iatrogenic arterial injury has become the predominant cause of pseudoaneurysm formation. The highest incidence of iatrogenic pseudoaneurysm formation is observed in the common femoral artery as a result of inadequate seal of the arterial puncture site following catheterisation procedures. It is reported that femoral pseudoaneurysms occur in up to 0.2% of diagnostic and 8% of interventional procedures.[2] Approach to the management of a pseudoaneurysm depends on its anatomical location. This chapter will focus primarily on the management of iatrogenic femoral pseudoaneurysms, with an overview of other peripheral and visceral iatrogenic pseudoaneurysms.

2. Femoral iatrogenic pseudoaneurysms

2.1. General considerations

Factors which may increase the risk of iatrogenic femoral pseudoaneurysm formation after femoral catheterisation can be broadly categorised into procedural or patient factors. 'Procedural' factors include low femoral puncture, inadvertent catheterisation of the superficial femoral artery or profunda femoris artery, interventional rather than diagnostic procedures, and inadequate compression following removal of the sheath. 'Patient' factors include obesity and the need for anticoagulation post-procedure.[2]

Patients with femoral pseudoaneurysms typically present with pain and swelling of the affected groin, along with a palpable mass which may be pulsatile with a thrill or bruit.[1] Clinical diagnosis can usually be made in slim patients, but can be difficult in those who are obese, where a high index of suspicion is required to prompt further investigation. Small pseudoaneurysms may resolve spontaneously without intervention. Pseudoaneurysms which persist may enlarge and lead to complications related to compression of the adjacent femoral vein, nerve, and overlying skin. This can lead to leg swelling, deep vein thrombosis, compressive neuropathy and skin necrosis. Although rare, pseudoaneurysms may also expand and eventually rupture.[3]

2.2. Diagnosis

Duplex ultrasonography (DUS) is the modality of choice for diagnosis of femoral pseudoaneurysms, particularly in centres with a dedicated vascular ultrasound laboratory.[4] DUS has been reported to have a sensitivity of 94% and a specificity of 97% in the detection femoral pseudoaneurysms.[5] Compared to other imaging techniques, DUS is safe and non-invasive. It can also be performed at the bedside. Clear views of the femoral vessels and associated pathology can be achieved rapidly in experienced hands. Another advantage of DUS is that definitive treatment (discussed later) can be performed in the same session.

On DUS, a pseudoaneurysm appears as a hypoechoic sac adjacent to the affected artery, with colour flow observed within it. Thrombus may be identified within part of the sac. The hallmark of diagnosis is the demonstration of a neck communicating between the sac and the affected artery, with a 'to-and-fro' waveform.[1] The 'to' representing blood flow into the pseudoaneurysm and the 'fro' representing blood flow out of the pseudoaneurysm. Waveform analysis of the affected artery is useful to establish a baseline for subsequent comparison. The adjacent vein should be inspected for compression or the presence of thrombus.

Computed Tomography Angiography (CTA) is another effective diagnostic modality, particularly in centres without ready access to vascular ultrasound services. It is also useful in cases where duplex ultrasound findings are equivocal or the anatomy is not well defined.[2] CTA allows accurate assessment of the pseudoaneurysm, its surrounding structures, arterial inflow and distal run-off to the leg. Drawbacks of CTA include radiation exposure (of particular concern in younger patients) and use of iodinated contrast agents (with risk of anaphylaxis and nephropathy).[6] Use of contrast is important to establish that active flow is present within the pseudoaneurysm cavity, which would be otherwise indistinguishable from a haematoma. Patients with mild renal impairment can be pre-hydrated before a CTA to minimise the risk of nephropathy. In those with moderate to severe renal impairment, alternative imaging should be considered.[6]

Magnetic Resonance Angiography (MRA) has emerged as an alternative to CTA in recent years. Gadolinium-enhanced MRA allows 3D visualisation of the pseudoaneurysm and surrounding structures. Problems with the technique include availability, time duration and cost. In patients with allergies to iodinated contrast, MRA is a potential alternative imaging technique.[1] Gadolinium-based agents are also associated with the rare complication of nephrogenic systemic fibrosis in patients with impaired renal function which should be considered as a relative contra-indication.[6]

2.3. Approach to management

A proportion of iatrogenic femoral pseudoaneurysms will resolve spontaneously without any form of intervention. An accepted approach is to monitor small (less than 3cm), stable, asymptomatic pseudoaneurysms, as the majority of them will thrombose within 4 weeks.[7] In one large series of small (<3cm) pseudoaneurysms, Toursarkissian *et al* reported a rate of spontaneous thrombosis of ~90% at 60 days of follow-up.[7] However, the need for regular follow-up resulting in possible delayed discharge from the hospital, and difficulty in patients reducing their activity while awaiting pseudoaneurysm resolution, has led to the early active management of most pseudoaneurysms.[2] An exception may be for very small (<1cm), stable, asymptomatic pseudoaneurysms, which could be managed conservatively with repeat imaging at one week after diagnosis to see if spontaneous thrombosis has occurred. In addition, spontaneous thrombosis of the pseudoaneurysm may be less likely in patients who are fully anticoagulated or receiving combination antiplatelet therapy, where active management is preferred.

Traditionally, most iatrogenic femoral pseudoaneurysms requiring intervention were treated with open surgical repair. With the increasing availability of DUS during the 1990s, less invasive treatment options using DUS-guidance gained popularity. These methods included ultrasound-guided compression (UGC) and percutaneous ultrasound-guided thrombin injection (UGTI). [8,9]

Open surgical repair (OSR) has traditionally been considered the 'gold standard' treatment for iatrogenic femoral pseudoaneurysms, as the arterial defect is repaired definitively. Principle steps of OSR involve obtaining proximal and distal control of the affected artery, evacuating the aneurysm sac and repairing the defect in the arterial wall (either by primary or patch closure).[10] Complications of OSR include blood loss and infection. Other major adverse events such as myocardial infarction or death are recognised. In high cardiac risk patients, OSR may be performed under local or regional anaesthesia. Recovery time and inpatient stay may be prolonged following OSR.

The advent of less invasive treatment strategies utilising ultrasound (discussed later), have led to a paradigm shift in treatment strategies. OSR is now typically reserved for emergency situations such as rapidly expanding pseudoaneurysms, ruptured pseudoaneurysms, pseudoaneurysms causing mass effect (with overlying skin ischaemia or neurovascular compromise), or when other treatment options have failed.[11] Infective complication of iatrogenic femoral pseudoaneurysms are less common but represent a distinct entity which require open surgical treatment over other interventional techniques and will be considered later in this chapter.

2.3.1. Ultrasound-Guided Compression

Ultrasound-Guided Compression (UGC) of pseudoaneurysms to induce thrombosis of the aneurysm sac was proposed as an alternative to surgery by Fellmeth et al in 1991.[8] Principles of UGC involve locating the aneurysm sac using the ultrasound transducer and applying enough pressure to stop flow within the sac, but maintain flow in the affected artery.[5] Flow within the sac is reassessed at 10 - 20 minute intervals until thrombosis is achieved.[1] Unfortunately, efficacy of this technique is limited, with success rates between 62% - 86%.[1,2] Compression times can also be lengthy. This occupies vascular ultrasound laboratory resources and can be uncomfortable for both the patient and clinician.[9] Other problems include incompressible pseudoaneurysms, limited success in patients being treated with anticoagulants & some early recurrences.[9] Despite this, before other minimally invasive treatment options were available, Perkins et al reported that UGC reduced the need for open surgery by about 50%, avoiding the associated risks of surgery in these patients.[9]

2.3.2. Ultrasound-Guided Thrombin Injection

Ultrasound-Guided Thrombin Injection (UGTI) of pseudoaneurysms is a technique first described by Kang et al in 1998.[12] The technique involves needle infiltration of the aneurysm sac using ultrasound guidance and injection of thrombin to induce thrombosis of the cavity. Previously published studies have documented rates of thrombosis between 86 - 100% (the majority successful on the first attempt).[2] The procedure has the advantage of being relatively quick and simple. The most serious complication of UGTI is distal arterial embolisation, which is a relatively rare outcome (less than 2% in reported series). If this occurs, intra-arterial thrombolysis may be undertaken.[13]

At the Oxford University Hospitals, UGTI has been used as first-line therapy for the treatment of iatrogenic femoral pseudoaneurysms. Between August 2005 and July 2011, 94 patients underwent UGTI for treatment of iatrogenic pseudoaneurysms. Patients were included in a prospective registry and underwent follow up DUS examination to assess treatment efficacy. 97% of pseudoaneurysms suitable for UGTI were successfully treated by this technique, avoiding the risks associated with surgical repair. 91.1% of treatments were successful on the first attempt, and no significant complications were recorded.

In our experience, we have found UGTI to be a simple, quick and safe technique for the treatment of suitable pseudoaneurysms. For small pseudoaneurysms (<1cm), a repeat DUS was performed one week later to see if spontaneous thrombosis had occurred. Pseudoaneurysms with a neck width >1cm were not treated by this method, as wide necks may be related to higher risk of thromboembolic complications.[14] Given the availability of DUS in most major vascular surgery units, UGTI should be the treatment of choice for all suitable iatrogenic pseudoaneurysms.

2.4. Technique of UGTI

Our unit has adapted the original technique for UGTI described by Kang et al for the treatment of suitable femoral iatrogenic pseudoaneurysms.[12] Each procedure is performed by a vascular surgeon (or senior surgical fellow), together with a specialist vascular ultrasonographer. The patient is placed in the supine position. The ultrasonographer uses B-mode and colour flow imaging to define the pseudoaneurysm. As a baseline, pre-procedure imaging of adjacent major vessels (e.g. common femoral artery and vein) is performed. 500 IU of lyophilised human thrombin is dissolved in 1ml calcium chloride solution. This is drawn into a 2ml syringe and a 22 gauge spinal needle is attached.

A safe angle of approach to the aneurysm sac is confirmed by the ultrasonographer and vascular surgeon. The area of skin puncture is prepared with chlorhexidine solution. The ultrasonographer provides a constant good view of the pseudoaneurysm using B-mode imaging while the needle is advanced slowly into the pseudoaneurysm cavity. The needle tip is positioned away from the neck of the pseudoaneurysm, but within a flowing component of the sac. Appropriate positioning within the sac is confirmed by the ultrasonographer using multiple views. Once the ultrasonographer and vascular surgeon are satisfied with the needle position, thrombin injection is performed. On occasions, the needle tip may be difficult to identify on ultrasound and a 20 gauge spinal needle is used to improve visualisation.

Thrombin injection is then performed slowly under constant colour flow imaging to observe thrombosis of the aneurysm sac. When colour flow within the cavity stops completely, injection is ceased. It is uncommon for us to require more than **0.25ml** of thrombin solution to achieve thrombosis, even for relatively large pseudoaneurysms. Another way of ensuring controlled injection of thrombin is to administer small (e.g. 0.125ml) aliquots of solution at a time whilst assessing colour flow within the aneurysm sac.

All patients are followed up at one week with repeat duplex ultrasound. Further injections may be undertaken at this stage if deemed appropriate. We advise caution and consideration of alternative treatment if more than two injections are required.

2.5. Infected femoral pseudoaneurysms

Infected femoral pseudoaneurysms are more commonly seen in the intravenous drug using (IVDU) population, arising from repeated non-sterile needle groin punctures as part of the pursuit of easy peripheral venous access. However, it may also complicate iatrogenic pseudoaneurysms. Clinical presentation mirrors that for non-infected femoral pseudoaneurysms, with the added serious complication of infection. The 'aneurysmal abscess' carries with it a significant risk of sepsis, rupture, limb loss and death.[15] Diagnosis can be made by DUS, but direct DUS imaging can be challenging due to inflammation and even gas. CTA avoids these problems, and can give an appreciation of the extent of inflammation/infection.

Primary repair is not recommended as appropriate surgical management by some authors because the ongoing infection and destruction of the arterial wall usually results in secondary haemorrhage and infection.[15] Ligation and excision of the infected artery and pseudoaneurysm, with aggressive debridement of surrounding infected tissue is the preferred approach. There is debate among vascular surgeons regarding whether a bypass procedure is required during the same operation.[15]

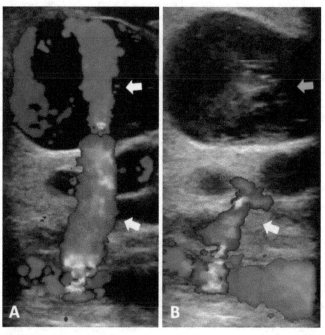

Figure 1. Panel A- DUS of femoral pseudoaneurysm demonstrating "to and fro" flow (yellow arrow) between the native artery and the pseudoaneurysm via the neck. There is colour signal in the pseudoaneurysm (white arrow) representing active blood flow. Panel B: Thrombosed pseudoaneurysm following UGTI. The pseudoanerusym sac now contains newly formed thrombus (blue arrow). Note the residual blood flow within the pseudoaneurysm neck after thrombosis of the pseudoaneurysm sac.

In our experience, ligation and excision of the infected artery and pseudoaneurysm, with aggressive debridement of surrounding infected tissue is well tolerated overall. This also avoids extended procedure times and potential complications associated with infection of bypass grafts. A recent review publication by Georgiadis et al showed an early occurrence of rest pain in 10.8% of patients and early risk of amputation in 5.7% of patients. Triple ligation (for pseudoaneurysms occurring at the common femoral bifurcation) likely results in worse outcomes for patients than single ligation.[15] In these patients, we advocate close monitoring of the affected limb in the immediate post-operative period and consideration for immediate extra-anatomical bypass if signs of limb-threatening ischemia develop.

2.6. Other peripheral iatrogenic pseudoaneurysms

In addition to femoral pseudoaneurysms, the most common sites for iatrogenic pseudoaneurysm formation are the brachial artery and popliteal artery. As with femoral iatrogenic pseudoaneurysms, most peripheral iatrogenic pseudoaneurysms occur following catheterisation of the affected artery. Clinical features will vary depending on the location and size of the pseudoaneurysm. Symptoms and signs will relate to the pseudoaneurysm itself and its effects on neighbouring structures. For example, brachial pseudoaneurysms often cause pain and swelling in the cubital fossa, along with a palpable mass. The mass may be pulsatile with a thrill or bruit. Compression of the adjacent brachial veins or median nerve can occur, as well as ischaemic compromise of the overlying skin. Arm swelling, deep vein thrombosis, compressive neuropathy, skin necrosis and rupture are also potential complications. Similarly, DUS is the modality of choice for diagnosis of other peripheral pseudoaneurysms, particularly in centres with a dedicated vascular ultrasound laboratory. CTA is best relied on in centres without ready access to vascular ultrasound services, in cases where duplex ultrasound findings are equivocal or the anatomy is not well defined.

The options available for management of peripheral pseudoaneurysms are the same as for femoral pseudoaneurysms. Given easy percutaneous access to the peripheries, UGTI should be the treatment of choice for all suitable iatrogenic peripheral pseudoaneurysms. Published series have reported successful outcomes of UGTI with pseudoaneurysms involving the femoral, popliteal, tibial, axillary, brachial and radial arteries.[16] Radial artery iatrogenic pseudoaneurysms following arterial line insertion in critical care settings can be better treated with radial artery ligation if there is clinically good perfusion via the ipsilateral ulnar artery.

Carotid artery pseudoaneurysms are a rare subset of pseudoaneurysms. Carotid aneurysms make up less than 1% of all carotid pathologies, and of these, roughly 1 in 3 are pseudoaneurysms.[13] In modern practice, the more common causes include inadvertent catherisation during attempted internal jugular vein central line placement, trauma (blunt or penetrating), and pseudoaneurysm formation in the anastomotic suture line following carotid endarterectomy. Local infection (e.g. TB, syphilis) causing pseudoaneurysm formation is rarely seen these days.

A pulsatile neck mass is the most common clinical presentation, followed by neurological symptoms such as TIA, stroke and Horner's syndrome.[13] Diagnosis can again be made by duplex ultrasound, however, with the possibility of endovascular intervention, CTA is best to define aortic arch anatomy and suitability for endovascular repair. The potential severe sequelae of carotid pseudoaneurysms mandates surgical intervention. Given small numbers, only case series data is available for different types of carotid aneurysm repair, with only a small subset of these comprising pseudoaneurysms. Open surgical intervention includes resection and patch angioplasty, resection and interposition grafting, and ligation.[13] The latter should be considered a last resort. Surgical reconstruction of all types of carotid aneurysm is associated with a combined stroke and mortality rate of about 10%.[17]

Endovascular interventions include covered stent grafts, bare stenting with trans-stent coiling, autogenous vein covered stents, and endovascular balloon occlusions.[13] Outcome data is limited to case series, but the data is promising. In a large single-centre series spanning 20 years, Zhou et al report that endovascular intervention is an effective alternative to open surgery, particularly for patients with high surgical risk or distally located aneurysms that preclude a safe surgical approach.[13]

2.7. Visceral iatrogenic pseudoaneurysms

Iatrogenic pseudoaneurysms arising from the thoraco-abdominal aorta and other visceral branches have all been reported. These are typically the complications of prior surgery (vascular or non-vascular) or endovascular intervention of arterial or venous pathologies.[18-21] Patients with visceral iatrogenic pseudoaneurysms may remain chronically asymptomatic with detection only after investigation for other complaints. Alternatively, presentation may be with local compressive symptoms, or even rupture. Endovascular treatment in the form of direct thrombin injection [22], coiling [23], occlusion devices [24], and endograft stenting [25,26] have all been described and often considered be first line option of treatment in most cases [27,28]. Open surgical repair of visceral iatrogenic pseudoaneurysms can be challenging, especially when in a previously exposed surgical field. Although there has been increasing utilization of endovascular techniques for the treatment of visceral iatrogenic pseudoaneurysms, there remains a clear role for OSR in selected situations, such as when local mass effect of pseudoaneurysms requires concurrent treatment.[27]

3. Conclusion

The incidence of iatrogenic pseudoaneurysms is increasing as a result of progressive uptake of percutaneous arterial interventions for cardiovascular disease and the increased use of combination antiplatelet therapy. Femoral iatrogenic pseudoaneurysms represent the most common form of this pathology, but the incidence of other peripheral / visceral pseudoaneurysms is also likely to increase in the future. In experienced hands, thrombin injection under DUS guidance can offer prompt resolution of the pathology. However, no large randomized trials to date have definitively addressed the efficacy of this treatment technique. Physicians should be aware of the potential for pseudoaneurysm formation following percutaneous arterial interventions, and be familiar with the clinical findings and potential treatment options.

Author details

Charles P.E. Milne and Regent Lee
Oxford Regional Vascular Unit, John Radcliffe Hospital, Oxford, UK

Ashok I. Handa*
Oxford Regional Vascular Unit, John Radcliffe Hospital, Oxford, UK
Nuffield Department of Surgical Sciences, John Radcliffe Hospital, Oxford, UK

* Corresponding Author

Acknowledgement

This work is funded by the Nuffield Department of Surgical Sciences.

Regent Lee is a Lumley Surgical Research Fellow and Foundation of Surgery Research Scholar with the Royal Australian College of Surgeons.

4. References

[1] Saad NE, Saad WE, Davies MG, Waldman DL, Fultz PJ, Rubens DJ. Pseudoaneurysms and the role of minimally invasive techniques in their management. Radiographics 2005;25 Suppl 1:S173-89.

[2] Ahmad F, Turner SA, Torrie P, Gibson M. Iatrogenic femoral artery pseudoaneurysms-- a review of current methods of diagnosis and treatment. Clin Radiol 2008;63:1310-6.

[3] De Raet J, Vandekerkhof J, Baeyens I. Ruptured femoral pseudo-aneurysm through the skin: a rare vexing complication following aortobifemoral reconstruction. Acta Chir Belg 2006;106:420-2.

[4] Middleton WD, Dasyam A, Teefey SA. Diagnosis and treatment of iatrogenic femoral artery pseudoaneurysms. Ultrasound Q 2005;21:3-17.

[5] Morgan R, Belli AM. Current treatment methods for postcatheterization pseudoaneurysms. J Vasc Interv Radiol 2003;14:697-710.

[6] Thomson K. Safe use of radiographic contrast media. Australia Prescriber 2010; :29-33.

[7] Toursarkissian B, Allen BT, Petrinec D et al. Spontaneous closure of selected iatrogenic pseudoaneurysms and arteriovenous fistulae. J Vasc Surg 1997;25:803-8; discussion 808-9.

[8] Fellmeth BD, Roberts AC, Bookstein JJ et al. Postangiographic femoral artery injuries: nonsurgical repair with US-guided compression. Radiology 1991;178:671-5.

[9] Perkins JM, Gordon AC, Magee TR, Hands LJ. Duplex-guided compression of femoral artery false aneurysms reduces the need for surgery. Ann R Coll Surg Engl 1996;78:473-5.

[10] Cronenwett J, editor Rutherford's Vascular Surgery. 7th ed: Saunders Elsevier: Philadelphia, 2010.

[11] Brummer U, Salcuni M, Salvati F, Bonomini M. Repair of femoral postcatheterization pseudoaneurysm and arteriovenous fistula with percutaneous implantation of endovascular stent. Nephrol Dial Transplant 2001;16:1728-9.

[12] Kang SS, Labropoulos N, Mansour MA, Baker WH. Percutaneous ultrasound guided thrombin injection: a new method for treating postcatheterization femoral pseudoaneurysms. J Vasc Surg 1998;27:1032-8.

[13] Zhou W, Lin PH, Bush RL et al. Carotid artery aneurysm: evolution of management over two decades. J Vasc Surg 2006;43:493-6; discussion 497.

[14] Edgerton JR, Moore DO, Nichols D et al. Obliteration of femoral artery pseudoaneurysm by thrombin injection. Ann Thorac Surg 2002;74:S1413-5.

[15] Georgiadis GS, Lazarides MK, Polychronidis A, Simopoulos C. Surgical treatment of femoral artery infected false aneurysms in drug abusers. ANZ J Surg 2005;75:1005-10.

[16] Friedman SG, Pellerito JS, Scher L, Faust G, Burke B, Safa T. Ultrasound-guided thrombin injection is the treatment of choice for femoral pseudoaneurysms. Arch Surg 2002;137:462-4.

[17] El-Sabrout R, Cooley DA. Extracranial carotid artery aneurysms: Texas Heart Institute experience. J Vasc Surg 2000;31:702-12.

[18] Skourtis G, Bountouris I, Papacharalambous G et al. Anastomotic pseudoaneurysms: our experience with 49 cases. Ann Vasc Surg 2006;20:582-9.

[19] Monney P, Pellaton C, Qanadli SD, Jeanrenaud X. Aortic pseudo-aneurysm caused by complete dehiscence of the left coronary artery 7 years after a composite mechanical-valved conduit aortic root replacement (Bentall operation). Eur Heart J 2012;33:60.

[20] Putterman D, Niman D, Cohen G. Aortic pseudoaneurysm after penetration by a Simon nitinol inferior vena cava filter. J Vasc Interv Radiol 2005;16:535-8.

[21] Konia M, Uppington J, Moore P, Liu H. Ascending aortic pseudoaneurysm: a late complication of coronary artery bypass. Anesth Analg 2008;106:767-8.

[22] Schellhammer F, Steinhaus D, Cohnen M, Hoppe J, Modder U, Furst G. Minimally invasive therapy of pseudoaneurysms of the trunk: application of thrombin. Cardiovasc Intervent Radiol 2008;31:535-41.

[23] Moneley D, Johnston KW, Tan KT, G O. Endovascular Treatment of an Iatrogenic Visceral Aortic Segment Aneurysm Following a Translumbar Vertebral Biopsy. EJVES Extra 2008;15:39-41.

[24] Sharma RP, Shetty PC, Burke TH, Shepard AD, Khaja F. Treatment of false aneurysm by using a detachable balloon. AJR Am J Roentgenol 1987;149:1279-80.

[25] Medina CR, Indes J, Smith C. Endovascular treatment of an abdominal aortic pseudoaneurysm as a late complication of inferior vena cava filter placement. J Vasc Surg 2006;43:1278-82.

[26] Pasklinsky G, Gasparis AP, Labropoulos N et al. Endovascular covered stenting for visceral artery pseudoaneurysm rupture: report of 2 cases and a summary of the disease process and treatment options. Vasc Endovascular Surg 2008;42:601-6.

[27] Kapoor BS, Haddad HL, Saddekni S, Lockhart ME. Diagnosis and management of pseudoaneurysms: an update. Curr Probl Diagn Radiol 2009;38:170-88.

[28] Keeling AN, McGrath FP, Lee MJ. Interventional radiology in the diagnosis, management, and follow-up of pseudoaneurysms. Cardiovasc Intervent Radiol 2009;32:2-18.

Permissions

The contributors of this book come from diverse backgrounds, making this book a truly international effort. This book will bring forth new frontiers with its revolutionizing research information and detailed analysis of the nascent developments around the world.

We would like to thank Dai Yamanouchi, MD, PhD, for lending his expertise to make the book truly unique. He has played a crucial role in the development of this book. Without his invaluable contribution this book wouldn't have been possible. He has made vital efforts to compile up to date information on the varied aspects of this subject to make this book a valuable addition to the collection of many professionals and students.

This book was conceptualized with the vision of imparting up-to-date information and advanced data in this field. To ensure the same, a matchless editorial board was set up. Every individual on the board went through rigorous rounds of assessment to prove their worth. After which they invested a large part of their time researching and compiling the most relevant data for our readers. Conferences and sessions were held from time to time between the editorial board and the contributing authors to present the data in the most comprehensible form. The editorial team has worked tirelessly to provide valuable and valid information to help people across the globe.

Every chapter published in this book has been scrutinized by our experts. Their significance has been extensively debated. The topics covered herein carry significant findings which will fuel the growth of the discipline. They may even be implemented as practical applications or may be referred to as a beginning point for another development. Chapters in this book were first published by InTech; hereby published with permission under the Creative Commons Attribution License or equivalent.

The editorial board has been involved in producing this book since its inception. They have spent rigorous hours researching and exploring the diverse topics which have resulted in the successful publishing of this book. They have passed on their knowledge of decades through this book. To expedite this challenging task, the publisher supported the team at every step. A small team of assistant editors was also appointed to further simplify the editing procedure and attain best results for the readers.

Our editorial team has been hand-picked from every corner of the world. Their multi-ethnicity adds dynamic inputs to the discussions which result in innovative outcomes. These outcomes are then further discussed with the researchers and contributors who give their valuable feedback and opinion regarding the same. The feedback is then collaborated with the researches and they are edited in a comprehensive manner to aid the understanding of the subject.

Apart from the editorial board, the designing team has also invested a significant amount of their time in understanding the subject and creating the most relevant covers. They scrutinized every image to scout for the most suitable representation of the subject and create an appropriate cover for the book.

The publishing team has been involved in this book since its early stages. They were actively engaged in every process, be it collecting the data, connecting with the contributors or procuring relevant information. The team has been an ardent support to the editorial, designing and production team. Their endless efforts to recruit the best for this project, has resulted in the accomplishment of this book. They are a veteran in the field of academics and their pool of knowledge is as vast as their experience in printing. Their expertise and guidance has proved useful at every step. Their uncompromising quality standards have made this book an exceptional effort. Their encouragement from time to time has been an inspiration for everyone.

The publisher and the editorial board hope that this book will prove to be a valuable piece of knowledge for researchers, students, practitioners and scholars across the globe.

List of Contributors

Igor Koncar, Nikola Ilic, Marko Dragas, Miroslav Markovic, Dusan Kostic and Lazar Davidovic
Clinic for Vascular and Endovascular Surgery, Serbian Clinical Centre, Serbia Medical Faculty, University of Belgrade, Serbia

Igor Banzic
Clinic for Vascular and Endovascular Surgery, Serbian Clinical Centre, Serbia

Luigi Chiariello, Paolo Nardi and Francesco Versaci
Cardiac Surgery Unit, Fondazione Policlinico Università Tor Vergata, Rome, Italy

Kiriakos Ktenidis and Argyrios Giannopoulos
1st Department of Surgery, Aristotle University of Thessaloniki, Greece

Jesus Barandiaran, Thomas Hall, Naif El-Barghouti and Eugene Perry
Department of Surgery, Scarborough General Hospital, UK

H.J.P. Fokkenrood, G.J. Lauret and J.A.W. Teijink
Department of Vascular Surgery, Catharina Hospital, Eindhoven, The Netherlands
CAPHRI Research School, Department of Epidemiology, Maastricht University, The Netherlands

H.J.M. Hendriks and R.A. de Bie
CAPHRI Research School, Department of Epidemiology, Maastricht University, The Netherlands

M.R.M. Scheltinga
Department of Vascular Surgery, Maxima Medical Centre, Veldhoven, The Netherlands

Charles P.E. Milne and Regent Lee
Oxford Regional Vascular Unit, John Radcliffe Hospital, Oxford, UK

Ashok I. Handa
Oxford Regional Vascular Unit, John Radcliffe Hospital, Oxford, UK
Nuffield Department of Surgical Sciences, John Radcliffe Hospital, Oxford, UK

Printed in the USA
CPSIA information can be obtained
at www.ICGtesting.com
JSHW011323221024
72173JS00003B/53

9 781632 420534